FOR REVIEW

March, 2014

S. EJAZ AHMED

Statistics for Biology and Health

Series Editors:
M. Gail
K. Krickeberg
J. Samet
A. Tsiatis
W. Wong

For further volumes:
http://www.springer.com/series/2848

Jong-Hyeon Jeong

Statistical Inference
on Residual Life

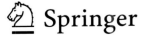 Springer

Jong-Hyeon Jeong
Department of Biostatistics
University of Pittsburgh
Pittsburgh, PA, USA

Supplementary material for this volume is available at www.springer.com.
Search for this title by print ISBN: 978-1-4939-0004-6

ISSN 1431-8776   ISSN 2197-5671 (electronic)
ISBN 978-1-4939-0004-6   ISBN 978-1-4939-0005-3 (eBook)
DOI 10.1007/978-1-4939-0005-3
Springer New York Heidelberg Dordrecht London

Library of Congress Control Number: 2013956615

Printed on acid-free paper

Springer is part of Springer Science+Business Media (www.springer.com)

To My Wife, Chang-Sook,
My Son, Michael,
and
My Daughter, Emily
for
All Your Love and Support

Preface

Life expectancy is an essential concept in the analysis of time-to-event data, which can be encountered in many research fields. Traditionally life expectancy has been defined as the mean residual lifetime, and much research effort has been devoted to the topic until recently. Potential asymmetric nature of time-to-event data also triggered researchers' interests in nonparametric approaches to inferring the remaining lifetimes in the mid-1980s, which has recently revived as a robust yet practical summary measure for censored survival data. In this book, we review the history and research achievements first in the topic of the mean residual lifetime and then elaborate on recent developments in statistical inference on the quantile residual lifetime.

Chapter 1 introduces the basic concepts needed to investigate the properties of the quantile (residual life) function such as almost sure convergence, strong law of large numbers, Brownian motion and bridge, empirical and quantile process, counting process martingale, and the check function. In Chap. 2, we briefly overview statistical methods developed to infer the mean residual life function. In Chap. 3, the quantile (residual life) function is defined and its properties are described, and recently developed inference methods are reviewed in detail. In Chap. 4, we elaborate on the extension of the results reviewed in Chap. 3 to the competing risks setting. In Chap. 5, we discuss some issues in inference on the quantile (residual life) function and review alternative methods based on the empirical likelihood and a Bayesian approach. In Chap. 6, we touch on a design aspect based on the quantile (residual life) function. In Appendix, we provide R codes that were written for the numerical examples throughout the book.

The targeted audience would be graduate students and researchers both in the academia and in the industry who are interested in learning theory and application of the quantile (residual life) function. Numerical examples in the book use small datasets, so that the readers can easily follow detailed calculations of the mathematical formulas, coupled with provided R codes. Real examples based on a dataset from a clinical trial are also included. At the end of each main chapter, future research directions are also suggested to stimulate researchers to move the field forward.

I would like to thank Professor David Oakes, who first introduced me to the topic of the proportional mean residual life model. My sincere thanks also go to Professors Jason Fine, Sin-Ho Jung, and Mai Zhou for our productive collaborations on the topics of competing risks analysis, quantile residual life inference, and empirical likelihood ratio inference, which had really broaden my knowledge in statistical theory and application. I would also like to thank the previous and current leadership of the Biostatistical Center for the National Surgical Adjuvant Breast and Bowel Project (NSABP), Professors Samuel Wieand, John Bryant, and Joseph P. Costantino, for their strong support for my methodological research. Finally I am very thankful to Professor Sally C. Morton, Chair of our department, for her constant encouragement and strong support while I was working on the book.

Pittsburgh, PA

Jong-Hyeon Jeong

Contents

Chapter 1

Introduction

In this chapter, we review some fundamental mathematical tools often used in development of probability and statistics theory, especially for the quantile (residual life) function, such as almost sure convergence, strong law of large numbers (SLLN), empirical processes, quantile processes, counting process martingale, Brownian motion, Brownian bridge, and the check function.

1.1 Almost Sure Convergence

The concept of almost sure convergence (a.s. convergence) is often used to prove uniform consistency of the empirical processes. Let us define Ω to be a sample space with its elements ω, and $\{X_n\}$ is a sequence of random variables defined on Ω. First, pointwise convergence of the sequence $\{X_n\}$ is defined such that the sequence of real numbers $\{X_n\}$ is convergent for all $\omega \in \Omega$. The a.s. convergence is a weaker convergence than the pointwise convergence in that it only requires the convergence of $\{X_n\}$ for a large enough subset of Ω with positive probability measure, not for all $\omega \in \Omega$. We denote the a.s. convergence of the sequence $\{X_n\}$ to its limit X as $X_n \to X$ a.s.

J.-H. Jeong, *Statistical Inference on Residual Life*,
Statistics for Biology and Health, DOI 10.1007/978-1-4939-0005-3_1,
© Springer Science+Business Media New York 2014

Example 1.1 (Statlec, The Digital Textbook, Lectures on Probability and Statistics, http://www.statlect.com/asconv1.htm). Suppose that we have the sample space $\Omega = [0, 1]$. For a sub-interval $[a, b] \in [0, 1]$, it is possible to build a probability measure P such that $P([a, b]) = b - a$ (Williams, 1991). Under this probability model, we have $P(\{w\}) = P([w, w]) = w - w = 0$, implying that a zero-probability is assigned to all the sample elements w. Now define a sequence of random variables as $\{X_n\} = 1$ if $\omega = 0$ and $1/n$ if $\omega \neq 0$. This implies that $X_n \rightarrow 0$ as $n \rightarrow \infty$ when $\omega \in (0, 1]$, while $X_n \rightarrow 1$ as $n \rightarrow \infty$ when $\omega = 0$. Therefore we can say that $X_n \rightarrow X = 0$ a.s. because it converges to 0 for all the sample points ω but 0, which is a zero-probability event. Often the sequence of random variables $\{X_n\}$ is also defined to converge a.s. to a constant c if and only if $P(|X_n - c| > \epsilon, \text{ i.o.}) = 0$ for all $\epsilon > 0$, where i.o. implies "infinitely often," or $\limsup_{n \rightarrow \infty} |X_n - c| = \inf_{n \rightarrow \infty} \left(\sup_{m \geq n} |X_n - c| \right) = 0$. That is, the almost sure convergence is equivalent to the statement that the probability of occurrence of an event of the absolute distance from the sequence X_n to the constant c remaining as large infinitely often becomes 0 as $n \rightarrow \infty$.

1.2   Strong Law of Large Numbers

The strong law of large numbers (SLLN) is also essential for proving the uniform consistency of the empirical processes.

Theorem 1 (SLLN). *Suppose that $X_1, X_2, \ldots, X_n$ is a random sample that has the cumulative distribution function $F(x)$. At a fixed value of x, define the indicator function $\delta_i = I(X_i \leq x) = 1$ if $X_i \leq x$ or 0 otherwise. If we define $F_n(x) = Y_n(x)/n$, where $Y_n(x) = \sum_{i=1}^n \delta_i$, as the empirical distribution function, then $F_n(x)$ converges a.s. to $p \equiv F(x)$.*

Proof: Note that at a fixed x, the indicator function δ_i is a Bernoulli random variable with mean p and variance $p(1 - p)$, and hence $E(\delta_i^4) = p < \infty$. Furthermore, by the Chebychev's inequality, for any ϵ, we have

$$P(|F_n(x) - p| > \epsilon) \leq \frac{E[F_n(x) - p]^4}{\epsilon^4} = \frac{E[Y_n(x) - np]^4}{(n\epsilon)^4}. \quad (1.1)$$

Since $Y_n(x)$ follows a binomial distribution with mean np, the 4th central moment $E[Y_n(x) - np]^4 = E[Y_n^4(x)] - 4(np)E[Y_n^3(x)] + 6(np)^2 E[Y_n^2(x)] - 4(np)^3 E[Y_n(x)] + (np)^4$ can be evaluated as $np(1 - p) + 3n(n - 2)p^2(1 - p)^2$ which is bounded by cn^2 as $n \to \infty$, where $c = 3p^2(1 - p)^2 < \infty$. Replacing $E[Y_n(x) - np]^4$ with cn^2 in inequality (1.1), we have

$$P(|F_n(x) - p| > \epsilon) \leq \frac{c}{n^2 \epsilon^4},$$

which implies

$$\sum_{n=1}^{\infty} P(|F_n(x) - p| > \epsilon) \leq \sum_{n=1}^{\infty} \frac{c}{n^2 \epsilon^4} < \infty.$$

Therefore by the Borel–Cantelli lemma (Borel, 1909; Cantelli, 1917), we finally have

$$P(|F_n(x) - p| > \epsilon, \text{i.o.}) = 0,$$

which implies that $F_n(x)$ converges to p a.s.

1.3 Brownian Motion and Brownian Bridge

In this section, we review a limiting process that plays crucial roles in deriving the limiting behavior of quantile (residual life) processes. The material being reviewed here is a summary from Ross (1985, Chap. 10).

1.3.1 Brownian Motion

The concept of the Brownian motion can be cast as a limiting behavior of the symmetric random walk. Under the symmetric random walk process, in each time unit, an object would be equally likely to take a unit step either to the left or to the right.

More formally, let us define $X(t)$ to be the position of the process, i.e. $X(t) = (\Delta x)(X_1 + X_2 + \ldots + X_{[t/\Delta t]})$, where $X_i = 1$ if the ith step of length Δx is to the left and -1 if it is to the right, and $[t/\Delta t]$ is the largest integer less than or equal to $t/\Delta t$. Note that $P(X_i = 1) = P(X_i = -1) = 1/2$, and hence $E[X(t)] = 0$ and $\text{Var}[X(t)] = (\Delta x)^2(t/\Delta t)$ since $E(X_i) = 0$ and $\text{Var}(X_i) = E(X_i^2) = 1$. For $c > 0$, letting $\Delta x = c\sqrt{\Delta t}$ gives $\text{Var}(X_i) = c^2t$ as $\Delta t \to 0$. By the central limit theorem, the process $X(t)$ follows a normal distribution with mean 0 and variance c^2t. In fact, under the simple random walk process, taking smaller and smaller steps (Δx) in smaller and smaller time intervals (Δt) leads to a Brownian motion as formally defined below.

Definiton 1.1. A stochastic process $\{X(t), t \geq 0\}$ is said to be a Brownian motion process (Wiener process) if

1. $X(0)=0$

2. $X(t), t \geq 0$ has stationary and independent increments. For example, the changes of value of the random walk in non-overlapping time intervals can be reasonably assumed to be independent and its distribution does not depend on t.

3. For all $t > 0$, $X(t)$ is normally distributed with mean 0 and variance c^2t, which only depends on the length of time that has passed since the previous time point. When $c = 1$, it is called standard Brownian motion.

Definiton 1.2. A stochastic process $X(t)$, $(t \geq 0)$, is called Gaussian or a normal process if $X(t_1), \ldots X(t_n)$ has a multivariate normal distribution for all $t_1, \ldots t_n$.

In general, the covariance process gives $\text{Cov}(X(t_1), X(t_2)) = \min(t_1, t_2)$ because

$$
\begin{aligned}
\text{Cov}(X(t_1), X(t_2)) &= \text{Cov}(X(t_1), X(t_1)+X(t_2)-X(t_1)) \\
&= \text{Cov}(X(t_1), X(t_1))+\text{Cov}(X(t_1), X(t_2)-X(t_1)) \\
&= \text{Cov}(X(t_1), X(t_1))=\text{Var}(X(t_1))=t_1, \qquad (1.2)
\end{aligned}
$$

when $t_1 \leq t_2$.

We will now show that the Brownian motion is the Gaussian process. Suppose $\{X(t), t \geq 0\}$ is a standard Brownian motion process with the probability density function

$$f_t(x) = \frac{1}{\sqrt{2\pi t}} \exp(-x^2/2t).$$

Note that for $t_1 < t_2 < \ldots < t_n$, the set of equalities $X(t_1) = x_1$, $X(t_2) = x_2, \ldots$, $X(t_n) = x_n$ is equivalent to $X(t_1) = x_1$, $X(t_2) - X(t_1) = x_2 - x_1, \ldots$, $X(t_n) - X(t_{n-1}) = x_n - x_{n-1}$. Since $X(t_1)$, $X(t_2) - X(t_1), \ldots$, $X(t_n) - X(t_{n-1})$ are independent and $X(t_k) - X(t_{k-1})$ is normally distributed with mean 0 and variance $t_k - t_{k-1}$ from (1.2), the joint probability density function is given by

$$
\begin{aligned}
f(x_1, x_2, \ldots, x_n) &= f_{t_1}(x_1) f_{t_2-t_1}(x_2-x_1) \ldots f_{t_n-t_{n-1}}(x_n-x_{n-1}) \\
&= \frac{\exp\left[-\frac{1}{2}\left\{\frac{x_1^2}{t_1} + \frac{(x_2-x_1)^2}{t_2-t_1} + \ldots + \frac{(x_n-x_{n-1})^2}{t_n-t_{n-1}}\right\}\right]}{(2\pi)^{n/2}\{t_1(t_2-t_1)\ldots(t_n-t_{n-1}\}^{1/2}}.
\end{aligned}
$$

$$(1.3)$$

Equation (1.3) implies that the random variables $X(t_1), X(t_2), \ldots,$ $X(t_n)$ follow a multivariate normal distribution. When $n = 2$, for example, the probability density function (1.3) reduces to

$$f(x_1, x_2) = \frac{\exp\left[-\frac{1}{2}\left\{\frac{x_1^2}{t_1} + \frac{(x_2-x_1)^2}{t_2-t_1}\right\}\right]}{(2\pi)\sqrt{t_1(t_2 - t_1)}},$$

which, after some manipulation, can be expressed as

$$f(x_1, x_2) = \frac{\exp\left[-\frac{1}{2(1-\rho^2)}\left\{\frac{x_1^2}{t_1} + \frac{x_2^2}{t_2} - 2\rho\left(\frac{x_1}{\sqrt{t_1}}\right)\left(\frac{x_2}{\sqrt{t_2}}\right)\right\}\right]}{(2\pi)\sqrt{t_1 t_2(1 - \rho^2)}},$$

where $\rho^2 = t_1/t_2$. This is the probability density function of a bivariate normal distribution with $(\mu_1, \mu_2, \sigma_1^2, \sigma_2^2, \rho) = (0, 0, t_1, t_2, \sqrt{t_1/t_2})$. From (1.2), the correlation coefficient ρ between $X(t_1)$ and $X(t_2)$ $(t_1 < t_2)$ is given by

$$
\begin{aligned}
\rho &= \frac{\mathrm{Cov}(X(t_1), X(t_2))}{\sqrt{\mathrm{Var}(X(t_1))\mathrm{Var}(X(t_2))}} \\
&= \frac{\min(t_1, t_2)}{\sqrt{t_1 t_2}} = \sqrt{\frac{t_1}{t_2}}.
\end{aligned}
$$

1.3.2   Brownian Bridge

The Brownian bridge is the Brownian motion process tied down both at 0 and 1. Denote $\{X(t), t \geq 0\}$ for the Brownian motion process and consider the process between 0 and 1 conditional on $X(1) = 0$. The conditional distribution of $X(s)$ given $X(t) = b$ when $s < t$ can be generally derived from

$$
\begin{aligned}
f_{s|t}(x|b) &= \frac{P[X(s) = x \text{ and } X(t) = b]}{P[X(t) = b]} \\
&= \frac{P[X(s) = x \text{ and } X(t) - X(s) = b - x]}{P[X(t) = b]} \\
&= \frac{P[X(s) = x]P[X(t) - X(s) = b - x]}{P[X(t) = b]} \\
&\propto \exp\left\{ -\frac{t(x - bs/t)^2}{2s(t - s)} \right\},
\end{aligned}
\tag{1.4}
$$

because $X(s)$ and $X(t) - X(s)$ are independent and normally distributed with the common mean 0 and variances s and $t-s$, respectively. This implies that the conditional distribution of $X(s)$ given $X(t) = b$ follows a normal distribution with mean $b(s/t)$ and variance $s(t - s)$. Applying this result to the Brownian bridge with a constraint of $X(1) = 0$, for any $s < t < 1$, we have $E\{X(s)|X(1) = 0\} = 0$ and the covariance process

$$
\begin{aligned}
\text{Cov}[(X(s), X(t))|X(1){=}0] &= E[X(s)X(t)|X(1){=}0] \\
&= E[X(t)E\{X(s)|X(t)\}|X(1){=}0] \\
&= E[X(t)(s/t)X(t)|X(1){=}0] \text{ by } (1.4) \\
&= (s/t)E[X(t)^2|X(1){=}0] \\
&= (s/t)\text{Var}[X(t)|X(1){=}0] \\
&= (s/t)t(1{-}t) \text{ by } (1.4) \\
&= s(1{-}t).
\end{aligned}
$$

Therefore, Brownian bridge is a Gaussian process with mean 0 and the covariance function $s(1 - t)$ $(0 \leq s < t \leq 1)$.

1.4 Empirical and Quantile Processes

1.4.1 Empirical Process

Suppose $X_1, X_2, \ldots, X_n$ is a random sample from a population with the distribution function $F(x)$. We first define $F_n(x) = (1/n) \sum_{i=1}^{n} I(X_i \leq t)$ as an empirical distribution function. By the SLLN, $F_n(x)$ converges a.s. to $F(x)$ at every fixed x, which can be extended to uniform consistency by the Glivenko–Cantelli theorem (Glivenko, 1933; Cantelli, 1933).

Theorem 2 (Glivenko–Cantelli). *If $X_1, X_2, \ldots$ are independently and identically distributed with the distribution function $F(x)$, then as $n \to \infty$*

$$\sup_x |F_n(x) - F(x)| \to 0 \ a.s.$$

Proof (Durrett, 1991, p. 56): Suppose that $F(x)$ is continuous. Let $x_{k,i} = \inf\{x : F(x) \geq i/k\}$ ($1 \leq i \leq k-1$), where k is defined such that

$$|F_n(x_{k,i,}) - F(x_{k,i,})| < 1/k,$$

for each i and a large n, by the strong law of the large numbers. This inequality also naturally holds for $x_{k,0} = -\infty$ and $x_{k,k} = \infty$. Therefore, for any $x \in (x_{k,i-1}, x_{k,i})$ and a large n, we have

$$F_n(x) \leq F_n(x_{k,i}) \leq F(x_{k,i}) + 1/k = F(x_{k,i-1}) + 2/k \leq F(x) + 2/k$$

and

$$F_n(x) \geq F_n(x_{k,i-1}) \geq F(x_{k,i-1}) - 1/k = F(x_{k,i}) - 2/k \geq F(x) - 2/k,$$

which implies that

$$\sup_x |F_n(x) - F(x)| \leq 2/k \to 0 \text{ as } n \to \infty.$$

For an independent sequence of random variables X_n of identically distributed real random variables, the Glivenko–Cantelli theorem allows the common distribution function F to be determined approximately (from the data), in the sense of almost sure uniform convergence (Bauer, 1995, p. 102).

Now we derive the limiting distribution of the empirical process $\sqrt{n}[F_n(x) - F(x)]$ through its inverse transformation. By the probability integral transformation, $\xi_i = F^{-1}(X_i)$ $(i = 1, 2, \ldots, n)$ would be a random sample following a uniform distribution between 0 and 1. Let us define the empirical distribution function of the uniform random variables ξ_i's as $G_n(t) = (1/n) \sum_{i=1}^{n} I(\xi_i \leq t)$ (Fig. 1.1a) and its corresponding true distribution function as $G(t)$. Note that both $nF_n(x)$ and $nG_n(F(x))$ follow the same binomial distribution $(n, F(x))$, because the events $X \leq x$ and $\xi \leq F(x)$ are equivalent and hence $P(X \leq x) = P(\xi \leq F(x)) = G((F(x)) = F(x)$. Therefore by setting $t = F(x)$, the process $\sqrt{n}[G_n(t) - t] = (1/\sqrt{n}) \sum_{i=1}^{n} [I(\xi_i \leq t) - t]$ $(0 \leq t \leq 1)$ can be defined as the uniform empirical process (Shorack and Wellner, 2009). This implies that the probablistic investigation of the process $\sqrt{n}[F_n(x) - F(x)]$ can be reduced to the uniform empirical process $\sqrt{n}[G_n(t) - t]$ $(0 \leq t \leq 1)$. It can be easily seen that $E[U_n(t)] = 0$ and, for $s < t$, the covariance process is given by

$$
\begin{aligned}
\mathrm{Cov}[U_n(s), U_n(t)] &= \mathrm{Cov}\left[\frac{1}{\sqrt{n}} \sum_{i=1}^{n} \{I(\xi_i \leq s) - s\}, \frac{1}{\sqrt{n}} \sum_{i=1}^{n} \{I(\xi_i \leq t) - t\} \right] \\
&= \mathrm{Cov}\left[I(\xi_i \leq s) - s, I(\xi_i \leq t) - t \right] \\
&= E\left[\{I(\xi_i \leq s) - s\}\{I(\xi_i \leq t) - t\} \right] \\
&= P(\xi_i \leq s) - t P(\xi_i \leq s) - s P(\xi_i \leq t) + ts \\
&= s - ts - st + ts = s(1 - t).
\end{aligned}
$$

Similarly, for $t < s$, we obtain $\mathrm{Cov}[U_n(s), U_n(t)] = t(1 - s)$, so that in general we have $\mathrm{Cov}[U_n(s), U_n(t)] = \min(s, t) - st$ $(0 \leq s, t \leq 1)$. This implies that under the assumptions for the Brownian bridge presented in Sect. 1.3 and by the ordinary multivariate central limit theorem, the uniform empirical process $U_n(t)$ converges to a Brownian bridge $B(t)$ (Doob, 1949; Donsker, 1951). This is equivalent to the statement that the original empirical process $\sqrt{n}[F_n(x) - F(x)]$ converges to a Brownian motion $B(F(x))$ with the covariance process of $F(\min(u, v)) - F(u)F(v)$.

1.4.2 Uniform Quantile Process

The asymptotic behavior of the uniform quantile process as a Brownian bridge will be useful later in Chap. 3 for deriving the asymptotic distribution of the quantile residual life function. Let us define $V_n(t) = \sqrt{n}[G_n^{-1}(t) - t]$ as the uniform quantile process, where $G_n^{-1}(t) = \inf\{x : G_n(x) \geq t\} = \xi_{n:i}$ for $(i-1)/n < t \leq i/n$ $(1 \leq i \leq n)$ (Fig. 1.1b), implying that the order statistic $\xi_{n:i}$ has its mean value of $i/(n+1)$ because it follows a Beta distribution $(i, n-i+1)$. By noting that

$$
\begin{aligned}
U_n\left(G_n^{-1}(t)\right) &= \sqrt{n}\left[G_n\left(G_n^{-1}(t)\right) - G_n^{-1}(t) + t - t\right] \\
&= -\sqrt{n}\left[G_n^{-1}(t) - t\right] + \sqrt{n}\left[G_n\left(G_n^{-1}(t)\right) - t\right],
\end{aligned}
$$

we can rewrite $V_n(t)$ as

$$
V_n(t) = -U_n\left(G_n^{-1}(t)\right) + \sqrt{n}\left[G_n\left(G_n^{-1}(t)\right) - t\right]. \tag{1.5}
$$

The second term in (1.5) is not equal to 0 when there is no jump (Fig. 1.1a, c), but it converges to 0 as the jump sizes get smaller as $n \to \infty$. Also note that $\sup_t |G_n(t) - t| = \sup_t |G_n^{-1}(t) - t|$ from Fig. 1.1a, b, and furthermore $\sup_t |G_n(t) - t| = \sup_t |G_n^{-1}(t) - t| \to 0$ a.s. by the Glivenko–Cantelli theorem (Shorack and Wellner, 2009, p. 95). This implies that both $G_n(t)$ and $G_n^{-1}(t)$ converge in distribution to $G(t) = t$ $(0 \leq t \leq 1)$, so that $V_n(t)$ converges to a Brownian bridge $-B(t)$.

1.5 Counting Process Martingale

We review the martingale and counting process theory here because it plays an important role in our development of the test statistics for the quantile residual life inference later.

1.5.1 Definition of Counting Process

First we define stochastic processes, or random processes, which are sequences of events governed by probabilistic laws (Karlin and Taylor, 1975), i.e. a time-indexed collection of random variables

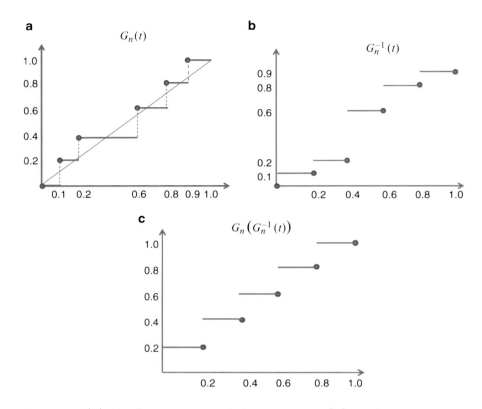

Fig. 1.1: (**a**) Uniform empirical distribution; (**b**) uniform quantile distribution; (**c**) inverse of uniform quantile distribution

or a mapping that assigns a time function to every outcome of points in the sample space. Suppose we have right-censored data with $X_i = \min(T_i, C_i)$ and $\delta_i = I(T_i \leq C_i)$, where T_i and C_i are potential failure time and censoring time, respectively. Let us define a counting process for a subject i as $N_i(t) = I(X_i \leq t, \delta_i = 1)$ $(i = 1, \ldots n)$ and $N(t) = \sum_{i=1}^{n} N_i(t)$. Then a stochastic process $N(t)$ is a counting process if

(i) $N(0) = 0$

(ii) $N(t) < \infty$ for all t with probability 1.

(iii) Sample paths are right-continuous and piecewise constant with jump size 1 when there are no ties.

Counting process theory for survival data has been developed by Aalen (1975), and well-known reference books on martingale and counting processes include Counting Processes and Survival Analysis (Fleming and Harrington, 1991), Statistical Models Based on Counting Processes (Andersen *et al.*, 1993), The Statistical Analysis of Failure Time Data (Kalbfleisch and Prentice, 2002, 2nd edn., Chap. 5), and Empirical Processes with Applications to Statistics (Shorack and Wellner, 2009, Chaps. 6–7).

1.5.2 Martingale

Martingale is a stochastic process where the best estimate of the future value conditional on the past, including the present, is the present value. The concept of martingale in probability theory was introduced by Paul Pierre Levy, and much of the original development of the theory was done by Joseph Leo Doob.

As a simple example of a martingale process, suppose a player tosses a *fair* coin with $p = q = 1/2$, and wins a dollar if heads come up and loses a dollar if tails come up. If we let $W_n = \sum_{i=1}^{n} X_i$ be his/her fortune at the end of n tosses, then $E(W_{n+1}|X_n, X_{n-1}, \ldots X_1) = \sum_{i=1}^{n} X_i + E(X_{n+1}) = W_n$, implying that the average fortune of the player at the $(n+1)^{th}$ toss is the same as his/her current fortune W_n, which is not affected by how (s)he arrived at this current fortune (a fair game). Depending on p, the game could be biased in favor of the player (submartingale) or against the player (supermartingale).

Let us define $\mathcal{F}_t$ as history, or filtration, of the counting process up to time t, and $\mathcal{F}_{t-}$ = history up to just before t. Note that $\mathcal{F}_t$ consists of knowledge of the pairs (T_i, δ_i) if $T_i \leq t$ and the knowledge that $T_i > t$ for the subjects still at risk at time t, as well as information on possibly time-dependent covariates at time t.

Definiton 1.3 (Martingale). $M(t)$ is a *martingale* if, for $s < t$

$$E(M(t)|\mathcal{F}_s) = M(s).$$

This definition is equivalent to

$$E(dM(t)|\mathcal{F}_s) = 0 \quad \text{for all} \quad t,$$

since

$$E(M(t)|\mathcal{F}_s) - M(s) = E(M(t) - M(s)|\mathcal{F}_s) = E\left[\int_s^t dM(u)|\mathcal{F}_s\right]$$
$$= \int_s^t E[E[dM(u)|\mathcal{F}_{u-}]|\mathcal{F}_s] = 0,$$

if $E[dM(t)|\mathcal{F}_{t-}] = 0$.

We can construct a martingale structure for the simple counting process $N(t)$ under censoring when T_i and C_i are independent. The conditional probability that a subject fails instantaneously at or after time t given that the subject did not fail prior to t can be expressed as

$$P(t \leq X_i < t + dt, \delta_i = 1|\mathcal{F}_{t-}) \approx \begin{cases} 0, & X_i < t, \\ h(t)dt, & X_i \geq t, \end{cases}$$

where $h(t)$ is the hazard function and the event $\{X_i \geq t\}$ would represent all information in the filtration $\mathcal{F}_{t-}$ in this case (without covariates) because it implies that X_i was neither censored nor occurred as an event prior to t. Here note that the identical failure time distribution is assumed for all observations (X_i, δ_i), which shares the common hazard function $h(t)$.

We have earlier defined the "individual" counting process $N_i(t) = I(X_i \leq t, \delta_i = 1)$ for the ith subject. Similarly let $Y_i(t) = I(X_i \geq t)$ denote an individual risk process. The increment of the individual counting process can be defined as $dN_i(t) = N_i((t+dt)^-) - N_i(t^-)$, which can be viewed as a conditional Bernoulli random variable because it can take only 0 or 1 with an instantaneous hazard rate $h(t)$ between t and $t + dt$ given that $X_i \geq t$. Therefore we have

$$E(dN_i(t)|\mathcal{F}_{t-}) = Y_i(t)h(t)dt \equiv \lambda_i(t)dt,$$

where $\lambda_i(t)$ is an individual intensity process that leads to the definition of the individual cumulative intensity process $\Lambda_i(t) = \int_0^t \lambda_i(s)ds$. Now for the "total" counting process $N(t) = \sum_{i=1}^n N_i(t)$, we have

$$
\begin{aligned}
E\{dN(t)|\mathcal{F}_{t-}\} &= E\{\sum_{i=1}^{n} dN_i(t)|\mathcal{F}_{t-}\} \\
&= \sum_{i=1}^{n} E\{dN_i(t)|\mathcal{F}_{t-}\} \\
&= Y(t)h(t)dt = \lambda(t)dt = d\Lambda(t),
\end{aligned}
$$

where $Y(t) = \sum_{i=1}^{n} Y_i(t)$ and $\Lambda(t) = \sum_{i=1}^{n} \int_0^t \lambda_i(s)ds = \sum_{i=1}^{n} \int_0^t Y_i(s)$
$h(s)ds = \int_0^t Y(s)h(s)ds$.

1.5.3 Basic Counting Process Martingale

The stochastic process $M(t) = N(t) - \Lambda(t)$ will be referred to as
the basic counting process martingale since

$$
\begin{aligned}
E(dM(t)|\mathcal{F}_{t-}) &= E(dN(t) - d\Lambda(t)|\mathcal{F}_{t-}) \\
&= E(dN(t)|\mathcal{F}_{t-}) - E(\lambda(t)dt|\mathcal{F}_{t-}) = 0.
\end{aligned}
$$

Note that $Y(t)$ is not random any more once all the history of
the process is known just prior to t. The function $\Lambda(t)$ is called
a compensator of the counting process $N(t)$, which is a smooth
(predictable) function as the conditional expectation of the counting process given $\mathcal{F}_{t-}$. It is well known that numerous statistics
frequently used to analyze censored survival data, such as Nelson–
Aalen estimator (Nelson, 1972; Aalen, 1978), Kaplan–Meier estimator (Kaplan and Meier, 1958), log-rank test statistic (Peto and
Peto, 1972), and partial likelihood function (Cox, 1975), can be
expressed as stochastic integrals with respect to the basic counting process martingale. Here the stochastic integral takes a form
of $\int_0^t K(s)dM(s)$, where $K(s)$ is a predictable process such as
$Y(t)$. Evaluation of the variance process of a stochastic integral
involves the predictable variation process of the basic counting
process martingale, denoted by $\langle M \rangle(t)$. The name of the predictable variation process comes from the fact that the increment
of the process $\langle M \rangle(t)$ is the variance of the increments of the
martingale $M(t)$ given the history just prior to t, which is identical to the variance of the increments of the counting process
$N(t)$ given the history just prior to t. Now to find the increment

of the process $\langle M \rangle (t)$, we start from the individual variation increment process $d \langle M_i \rangle (t)$. Because $d\Lambda_i(t)$ is predictable and $E\{dN_i(t)|\mathcal{F}_{t-}\} = d\Lambda_i(t)$, we have

$$
\begin{aligned}
d \langle M_i \rangle (t) &\equiv \mathrm{Var}\{dM_i(t)|\mathcal{F}_{t-}\} = E[\{dM_i(t)\}^2|\mathcal{F}_{t-}] \\
&= E[\{dN_i(t) - d\Lambda_i(t)\}^2|\mathcal{F}_{t-}] \\
&= E[\{dN_i(t)\}^2 - 2\{dN_i(t)\}\{\Lambda_i(t)\} + \{d\Lambda_i(t)\}^2|\mathcal{F}_{t-}] \\
&= E[\{dN_i(t)\}|\mathcal{F}_{t-}] - 2\Lambda_i(t)E\{dN_i(t)|\mathcal{F}_{t-}\} + d\Lambda_i(t)^2 \\
&= d\Lambda_i(t) - 2\{d\Lambda_i(t)\}^2 + \{d\Lambda_i(t)\}^2 \\
&= d\Lambda_i(t)\{1 - d\Lambda_i(t)\} \\
&= Y_i(t)h(t)dt\{1 - Y_i(t)h(t)dt\} \\
&= Y_i(t)h(t)dt\{1 - h(t)dt\} \\
&= Y_i(t)dH(t)\{1 - dH(t)\}, \quad\quad\quad (1.6)
\end{aligned}
$$

where $H(t) = \int_0^t h(s)ds$ is the cumulative hazard function. Since the individual martingale increments $dM_i(t)$ $(i = 1, 2, \ldots, n)$ are independent, we have the total variation increment process as

$$
\begin{aligned}
d \langle M \rangle (t) &= \mathrm{Var}\{dM(t)|\mathcal{F}_{t-}\} \\
&= \sum_{i=1}^n \mathrm{Var}\{dM_i(t)|\mathcal{F}_{t-}\} \\
&= \sum_{i=1}^n Y_i(t)dH(t)\{1 - dH(t)\} \\
&= Y(t)dH(t)\{1 - dH(t)\}.
\end{aligned}
$$

This implies that the predictable variation process of $M(t)$ is given by

$$
\langle M \rangle (t) = \int_{-\infty}^t Y(s)\{1 - \Delta H(s)\}dH(s).
$$

This also implies that the process $Q(t) = M^2(t) - \langle M \rangle (t)$ is a martingale because $E\{dQ(t)|\mathcal{F}_{t-}\} = E\{dM^2(t) - d \langle M \rangle (t)|\mathcal{F}_{t-}\} = 0$ and $\langle M \rangle (t)$ is the compensator for the square integrable martingale process $M^2(t)$.

Now the predictable variation process of stochastic integrals can be expressed as (Fleming and Harrington, 1991, Theorems 2.4.2 and 2.4.3)

$$\left\langle \int_0^t K(s)dM(s) \right\rangle = \int_0^t K(s)^2 d\langle M\rangle(s)$$
$$= \int_0^t K(s)^2 Y(s)\{1 - \Delta H(s)\}dH(s).$$

This implies that the variance of the stochastic integrals is the weighted sum of the variances of conditionally independent increments of the total basic martingale process $M(t)$.

1.5.4 Martingale Representation of the Kaplan–Meier Estimator

The Kaplan–Meier estimator can be defined via the Nelson–Aalen estimator of the cumulative hazard function, i.e.

$$\hat{S}(t) = \prod_{s=0}^{t}[1 - d\hat{H}(s)],$$

where $\hat{H}(t) = \int_0^t J(s)dN(s)/Y(s)$, where $J(s) = I(Y(s) > 0)$, is the Nelson–Aalen estimator for the cumulative hazard function. The Kaplan–Meier estimator itself cannot be expressed directly as a stochastic process with respect to the basic martingale, but $\hat{S}(t)/S(t) - 1$ can as follows (Fleming and Harrington, 1991, Theorem 3.2.3 and Corollary 3.2.1):

$$\hat{G}(t) \equiv \hat{S}(t)/S^*(t) - 1 = \int_0^t \frac{\hat{S}(s-)J(s)}{S^*(s)Y(s)}dM(s), \tag{1.7}$$

where $S^*(t) = \prod_{s=0}^{t}\{1 - J(s)dH(s)\}$ for a discrete case, which is assumed to approach asymptotically to $S(t)$ for all t. One can see that $\hat{G}(t)$ in Eq. (1.7) is a stochastic integral because $\hat{S}(s-)$, $J(s)$, $S^*(s)$, and $Y(s)$ are predictable at any given s. Therefore the predictable variation process of $\hat{G}(t)$ is given by

$$V_{\hat{G}}(t) = \langle \hat{G}\rangle(t) = \int_0^t \left\{ \frac{\hat{S}(s-)J(s)}{S^*(s)Y(s)} \right\}^2 d\langle M\rangle(s),$$

where $d\langle M\rangle(s) = Y(s)\{1 - \Delta H(s)\}dH(s)$. By replacing $H(s)$ with its estimate $\hat{H}(s) = \int_0^t \frac{J(s)}{Y(s)}dN(s)$, $S^*(s)$ with $\hat{S}(s) = \prod_{s=0}^t \{1 - d\hat{H}(s)\}$, and noting that $\hat{S}(s-)/\hat{S}(s) = \{1 - dJ(s)H(s)\}^{-1}$, we have the estimated variation process for $\hat{G}(t)$

$$V_{\hat{G}}(t) = \int_0^t \frac{dN(s)}{Y(s)\{Y(s) - \Delta N(s)\}}. \tag{1.8}$$

Since $\text{Var}[\hat{G}(t)] = \text{Var}[\hat{S}(t)]/\{S^*(t)\}^2$, the estimated variation process for $\hat{S}(t)$ is given by

$$\hat{V}_{\hat{S}}(t) \equiv \widehat{\text{Var}}\{\hat{S}(t)\} = \{\hat{S}(t)\}^2 \int_0^t \frac{dN(s)}{Y(s)\{Y(s) - \Delta N(s)\}},$$

which coincides with the Greenwood's formula (Greenwood, 1926).

To investigate the limiting behavior of the modified Kaplan–Meier process (1.7), we heuristically mention here Rebolledo's Martingale Central Limit Theorem (MCLT) (Shorack and Wellner, 2009, p. 262). The crucial assumptions for the MCLT (Kalbfleisch and Prentice, 2002, pp. 165–166) are (i) the stochastic integrals with appropriately standardized predictable functions (divided by n, for example) approach a limit as $n \to \infty$ and (ii) the influence of any single process is negligible in the limit (Fleming and Harrington, 1991, Lindberg condition, p. 207).

Theorem 3 (Martingale Central Limit Theorem (Reboll edo)). *If $M_n(t)$ is a martingale that satisfies the Lindberg condition and its predictable variation process $\langle M_n\rangle(t)$ converges in probability to some limiting value $V(t)$ as $n \to \infty$ for each t, where $V(t)$ is increasing and right-continuous with $V(-\infty) = 0$, then $M_n(t)$ converges to the Brownian motion $B(V(t))$ with its variance process of $V(t)$.*

For example, the modified Kaplan–Meier process in (1.7) is a martingale with its predictable variation process given in (1.8), which has the limiting value of $nV_G(t) = \int_0^t h(s)ds/y(s)$, where $y(s) = \lim_{n\to\infty} Y(s)/n$. Interestingly, this is the same predictable variation process as one for the Nelson–Aalen estimator. Therefore, from the MCLT, the process $\sqrt{n}[\hat{G}(t) - G(t)]$ converges weakly to the Brownian motion with the covariance process of $nV_G(\min(s,t))$, and hence the Kaplan–Meier process $\sqrt{n}[\hat{S}(t) - S(t)]$ converges weakly to the Brownian motion with the covariance process

$$nV_S(\min(s,t)) = S^2(\min(s,t)) \int_0^{\min(s,t)} \frac{h(u)du}{y(u)}.$$

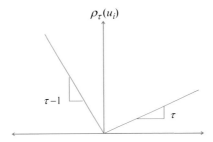

Fig. 1.2: A graph of the ρ-function, viewed as the loss function for the τ-quantile

1.6 Check Function

The estimating function for the quantile (residual life) function can be often expressed as the "check function" (Koenker and Bassett, 1978), which is briefly defined in this section. Let us consider a random sample of $X_1, X_2, \ldots, X_n$ from a population with its median $\theta_{\frac{1}{2}}$. By its definition, the sample median would minimize the sum of the absolute deviations of X_i's from itself, i.e. $\sum_{i=1}^n |X_i - \theta_{\frac{1}{2}}|$. Here the individual absolute deviation can be rewritten as

$$
\begin{aligned}
|X_i - \theta_{\frac{1}{2}}| &= (X_i - \theta_{\frac{1}{2}})I(X_i \geq \theta_{\frac{1}{2}}) - (X_i - \theta_{\frac{1}{2}})I(X_i < \theta_{\frac{1}{2}}) \\
&= (X_i - \theta_{\frac{1}{2}})[1 - I(X_i < \theta_{\frac{1}{2}})] - (X_i - \theta_{\frac{1}{2}})I(X_i < \theta_{\frac{1}{2}}) \\
&= 2u_i[1/2 - I(u_i < 0)] \\
&\equiv 2\rho_{\frac{1}{2}}(u_i),
\end{aligned}
\tag{1.9}
$$

where $u_i = X_i - \theta_{\frac{1}{2}}$. To find $\theta_{\frac{1}{2}}$ that minimizes $\sum_{i=1}^{n} \rho_{\frac{1}{2}}(u_i)$ from observed values of X_i's, taking the first derivative with respect to $\theta_{\frac{1}{2}}$ provides an estimating equation

$$\sum_{i=1}^{n} [1/2 - I(u_i < 0)] \equiv \sum_{i=1}^{n} \psi_{\frac{1}{2}}(u_i) = 0.$$

In general, for any $\tau-$quantile, the check function is defined as $\rho_{\tau}(u_i) = u_i[\tau - I(u_i < 0)]$, which can be interpreted as the loss function for the quantile of interest, analogous to the squared error loss for the mean (Fig. 1.2). In general, note that the absolute deviation function takes a form of $|Y - f(X)|$, where Y is the response variable and $f(X)$ is the systematic part of the model such as the median, the mean, or the regression function.

Chapter 2

Inference on Mean Residual Life-Overview

Statistical inference based on the remaining lifetimes would be intuitively more appealing than the popular hazard function defined as the risk of immediate failure, whose interpretation could be sometimes difficult to be grasped. For example, when an efficacy of a new drug is concerned, it would be more straightforward to explain it as "if one with the similar genetic and environmental background like you takes this drug, it is expected, on average, that it will prolong your remaining life years by 10 years" rather than simply saying "the average hazard reduction in the treatment group will be 25%." Common summary measures for the remaining lifetimes have been the mean and median residual lifetimes. This chapter presents a brief overview of statistical inference on the mean residual life, because the main focus of this book will be on the quantile residual life function.

We first define the mean residual life function and discuss the asymptotic properties of one-sample nonparametric estimator. Various regression models are then reviewed such as the proportional mean residual life model (Oakes and Dasu, 1990), the expectancy regression model (Chen and Cheng, 2006; Chen, 2007), the proportional scaled mean residual life model (Liu and Ghosh,

J.-H. Jeong, *Statistical Inference on Residual Life*,
Statistics for Biology and Health, DOI 10.1007/978-1-4939-0005-3_2,
© Springer Science+Business Media New York 2014

2008), and a general family of transformation models under the additive mean residual life structure (Sun and Zhang, 2009).

2.1   Mean Residual Life Function

The usage of mean residual life dates back to the third century A.D. (Deevey, 1947; Chiang, 1968; Guess and Proschan, 1985). Assuming that T is a continuous random variable with survival function $S(t)$, the mean residual life function is defined as the expected value of the remaining lifetimes after a fixed time point t, i.e.

$$
\begin{aligned}
e(t) &= E(T - t | T > t) \\
&= \frac{\int_t^\infty S(v)dv}{S(t)} \\
&= \frac{\int_t^\infty v f(v)dv}{S(t)} - t,
\end{aligned}
\tag{2.1}
$$

which exists for all t if and only if $e(0) = E(T)$ is finite (Oakes and Dasu, 2003). For example, for an exponential distribution with the probability density function $f(t) = \mu \exp(-\mu t)$, the mean residual life function is given as the mean of the distribution, i.e. $e(t) = 1/\mu$.

As succinctly summarized in McLain and Ghosh (2011), Hall and Wellner (1981, Proposition 2) provided a characterization theorem that gives the necessary and sufficient conditions for existence of the mean residual life function of a continuous nonnegative random variable:

(a) $e(t) \geq 0$ for all $t \geq 0$, and continuous,

(b) $e(t) + t$ is nondecreasing in t,

(c) if there exists a ω such that $e(\omega) = 0$, then $e(t) = 0$ for all $t \geq \omega$; otherwise, $\int_0^\infty e^{-1}(v)dv = \infty$.

The mean residual life function can be inverted to the survival function for more tractability by using the Inversion Formula (Gumbel, 1924; Cox, 1962, p. 128)

$$S(t) = \frac{e(0)}{e(t)} \exp\left\{ -\int_0^t \frac{dv}{e(v)} \right\}. \tag{2.2}$$

The variance formula for the mean residual life function, attributed by Hall and Wellner (1981) to Pyke (1965), can be derived as

$$\sigma(t) \equiv \operatorname{Var}(T - t | T > t) = \frac{\int_t^\infty e^2(v) f(v) dv}{S(t)}.$$

This formula also shows that $\sigma(t)$ is finite for all t if and only if $\sigma(0) = \operatorname{Var}(T)$ is finite. Hall and Wellner (1981) considered a family of the mean residual life function linear in t, i.e. $e(t) = at + b$ (Hall–Wellner family), which gives the survival function

$$S(t) = \left(\frac{b}{at + b} \right)_+^{1+1/a},$$

where the subscript $+$ implies that only the positive part of the expression in the parentheses is taken. Special cases of this family are a Pareto distribution, an exponential distribution, and a beta distribution for $a > 0$, $a = 0$, and $-1 < a < 0$, respectively (Oakes and Dasu, 2003).

2.2 One- and Two-sample Cases

For a random sample $T_1, T_2, \ldots, T_n$ from a distribution with the cumulative distribution function $F(t)$, and hence the survival function $S(t) = 1 - F(t)$, without censoring the natural one-sample nonparametric estimator for the mean residual life function at age t would be the sample mean of the residual lifetimes of the observations that exceed t, i.e.

$$\hat{e}(t) = \frac{\sum_{i=1}^n (T_i - t) I(T_i > t)}{\sum_{i=1}^n I(T_i > t)},$$

where $I(T_i > t) = 1$ if $T_i > t$ and 0 otherwise, so the denominator is the total number of observations that exceed t. Yang (1978) and Csörgö, Csörgö and Horváth (1986) showed that the process

$$Z_n(t) = \sqrt{n}[\hat{e}(t) - e(t)]$$

converges to a Gaussian process $Z(t)$ with 0 mean and covariance function

$$\text{Cov}[Z(s), Z(t)] = \frac{\sigma(\max(s,t))}{S(\min(s,t))}.$$

Yang (1978) noted that for $t > 0$, $\hat{e}(t)$ become slightly biased as $E[\hat{e}(t)] = e(t)[1 - F^n(t)]$, which, however, converges to $e(t)$ asymptotically (see also Gertsbakh and Kordonskiy, 1969).

Hall and Wellner (1981) and Bhattacharjee (1982) studied thoroughly on the mean residual life function, deriving necessary and sufficient conditions for an arbitrary function to be a mean residual life function. As mentioned above, Hall and Wellner (1981) also characterized a family of the mean residual life functions that are linear in age t. Guess and Proschan (1985) extensively reviewed both theory and application aspects of the mean residual life function. As they stated, for any distribution with a finite mean, the mean residual life function completely determines the distribution via the Inversion Formula as the probability density function, the moment generating function, or the characteristic function does. Bryson and Siddiqui (1969) defined various criteria for aging such as increasing failure rate (IFR) class, new better than used (NBU) class, decreasing mean residual life (DMRL) class, and new better than used in expectation (NBUE) class. Hollander and Proschan (1975) derived statistics to test the null hypothesis that the underlying failure distribution is exponential against the alternative hypothesis that it has a monotone mean residual life function. Chen *et al.* (1983) extended the Hollander–Proschan tests to censored survival data. Nair and Nair (1989) introduced the concept of the bivariate mean residual life function. Other related work in reliability theory also includes Watson and Wells (1961), Mute (1977), Bartholomew (1973), and Morrison and Schmittlein (1980). Berger, Boos, and Guess (1988) proposed a nonparametric test statistic to compare the mean residual life functions based on two independent samples.

2.3 Regression on Mean Residual Life

Analogous to Cox's proportional hazards model (Cox, 1972), Oakes and Dasu (1990) proposed the proportional mean residual life model

$$e_1(t; \theta) = \theta e_0(t), \tag{2.3}$$

where $\theta = \exp(\beta' z)$, β being a vector of regression coefficients and z a vector of covariates. Here $e_0(t)$ and $e_1(t; \theta)$ are the mean residual life function for the baseline and one adjusted for z, respectively. It seems that early literature on regression modeling for the mean residual life function has been revolving around the proportional mean residual life model. Therefore, we first review briefly existing statistical inference procedures under the proportional mean residual life model.

Applying the Inversion Formula in (2.2) twice under the model (2.3), we have

$$
\begin{aligned}
S_1(t; \theta) &= \frac{e_1(0; \theta)}{e_1(t; \theta)} \exp\left\{ -\int^t \frac{dv}{e_1(v; \theta)} \right\} \\
&= \frac{e_0(0)}{e_0(t)} \exp\left\{ -\frac{1}{\theta} \int^t \frac{dv}{e_0(v)} \right\} \\
&= S_0(t) \left(\frac{\int_t^\infty S_0(v) dv}{\mu_0} \right)^{1/\theta - 1},
\end{aligned}
\tag{2.4}
$$

where $\mu_0 = e_0(0)$ is the mean of the distribution at the origin.

Taking the first derivative of the middle line in (2.4) gives the probability density function

$$f_1(t; \theta) = -dS_1(t; \theta)/dt = \frac{\mu_0}{e_0^2(t)} \left\{ e_0'(t) + \frac{1}{\theta} \right\} \exp\left\{ -\frac{1}{\theta} \int_0^t \frac{dv}{e_0(v)} \right\}. \tag{2.5}$$

Once the baseline survival function is specified in (2.4) or the baseline mean residual life function is specified in (2.5), the maximum likelihood estimation method under the proportional mean residual life model can be readily applied to estimate the parameters for the baseline distribution and the proportionality parameter θ simultaneously, for both uncensored and censored survival data. Specifically, denoting C_i $(i = 1, \ldots, n)$ to be the random censoring time, $X_i = \min(T_i, C_i)$, and $\delta_i = I(T_i < C_i)$, the log-likelihood function will be given as

$$l(\theta; x_i) = \sum_{i=1}^{n} [\delta_i \log\{f_1(x_i; \theta)\} + (1 - \delta_i) \log\{S_1(x_i; \theta)\}].$$

For the uncensored case where the baseline distribution is completely known, Dasu (1991) and Oakes and Dasu (2003) showed that the score function per observation takes the form of

$$U(\theta) = \frac{d \log f(x; \theta)}{d\theta} = \frac{1}{\theta^2} \int_0^x \frac{dv}{e_0(v)} - \frac{1}{\theta\{1 + \theta e_0'(x)\}},$$

and hence the Fisher information is given by

$$I(\theta) = \frac{1}{\theta^2} \int_0^\infty \frac{S_1^2(v; \theta)}{e_1^2(v; \theta) f_1(v; \theta)} dv.$$

Therefore from the large sample theory, the asymptotic distribution of $\sqrt{n}(\hat{\theta} - \theta)$, where $\hat{\theta}$ is the maximum likelihood estimator of θ, follows a normal distribution with mean 0 and variance $I^{-1}(\theta)$.

For the semiparametric inference under the proportional mean residual life model, Oakes and Dasu (2003) proposed an estimator for θ for a binary covariate case, but its asymptotic behavior was not proved. Maguluri and Zhang (1994) modified the partial likelihood-based inference (Cox, 1972, 1975) by using the fact that for any stationary renewal process (Karlin and Taylor, 1975) the mean residual life function can be expressed as the reciprocal of the hazard function of the residual life distribution, but mainly for the uncensored case. Chen and Cheng (2005) and Chen et al. (2005) employed the counting process theory to develop a new inference procedure for censored survival data under the proportional mean residual life model. Their approach mimics the Cox partial score function, resulting in a closed form of the baseline mean residual life estimator and hence a regression coefficient estimator that resembles the maximum partial likelihood estimator.

Zhao and Qin (2006) applied an empirical likelihood ratio to construct the confidence regions for the regression parameters. Chan *et al.* (2012) considered inference on the proportional mean residual life model for right-censored and length-biased data. Chen and Wang (2013) proposed an estimation procedure via the augmented inverse probability weighting and kernel smoothing techniques under the proportional mean residual life model with missing at random.

For other regression models, Chen and Cheng (2006) and Chen (2007) proposed expectancy regression model where the mean residual life functions are additive, i.e.

$$e(t; z) = e_0(t) + \beta' z.$$

However, estimation under this model is subject to the constraint that $e(t; z) \geq 0$ for all z and $t \geq 0$, which is difficult to be satisfied, as noted in McLain and Ghosh (2011). Zhang *et al.* (2010) developed goodness-of-fit tests for this model. Liu and Ghosh (2008) proposed a proportional scaled mean residual life model that satisfies the first two characterization conditions (a) and (b),

$$e(t; z) = e_0\{t \exp(-\beta' z)\} \exp(\beta' z).$$

This model can be shown to be equivalent to the accelerated failure time model, but interpretation of β is not straightforward in terms of the mean residual life function. Sun and Zhang (2009) proposed the general family of semiparametric transformation models,

$$e(t; z) = g\{e_0(t) + \beta' z\},$$

for a transformation function $g(\cdot)$, which includes the proportional and additive mean residual life models as special cases, but they noted that the characterization condition (b) is still difficult to be met in general. Sun *et al.* (2011) extended this model to the case with time-dependent covariates under right censoring. McLain and Ghosh (2011) interestingly proposed two semiparametric estimators to estimate directly the mean residual life function adjusted for covariates. By using existing smoothing techniques, they estimated the adjusted survival functions first and plug them into the middle line in (2.1) to ensure that their estimators produce the mean residual life estimates that satisfy all of the characterization conditions (a)–(c). Their methods were applied to both proportional and additive mean residual life models.

In this chapter, a brief overview of statistical inference on the mean residual life function was presented. Major advantages of using the mean residual life function would be that it can be uniquely defined as long as the mean and variance of the distribution at the origin are defined, and that the proper statistical methods are well established in the literature and are expected to work nicely especially when the distribution of interest is symmetric. However, as first mentioned by Schmittlein and Morrison (1981), event-time data can be easily skewed, which might introduce biases in inference based on the center of the distribution. Parallel to the development of statistical methods in the topic of the mean residual life, there also has been vigorous research recently on the median or quantile residual life function. Starting from the next chapter, this book will be devoted to review recent developments in statistical inference on the quantile residual life function and to introduce new approaches where it is appropriate.

Chapter 3

Quantile Residual Life

As mentioned in Chap. 2, the mean residual life function is sensitive to outliers. In this chapter, as an alternative we consider the quantile residual life function, which is robust under any skewed distribution. We first review asymptotic theories of the quantile function and quantile residual life function and derive the quantile residual life process as a Brownian bridge. We also discuss parametric and nonparametric inferences on the quantile residual life function for one-sample, two-sample, and regression settings. Specifically, parametric inference based on the invariance property of the maximum likelihood estimator is outlined for one-sample and two-sample cases. For parametric regression, we consider a conditional log-linear regression on the residual lifetimes at a fixed time point and the maximum likelihood principles are also applied here. For parametric regression, we also review an invariance property of a certain family of distributions in their residual life distributions (Rao, Damaraju, and Alhumoud, 1993). For nonparametric inference for two-sample case and semiparametric regression, we mainly review the methods proposed by Jeong, Jung, and Costantino (2007) and Jung, Jeong, and Bandos (2009), respectively. We also present an alternative estimating equation to one proposed by Jung *et al.* (2009) by using the check function. For each numerical example

J.-H. Jeong, *Statistical Inference on Residual Life*,
Statistics for Biology and Health, DOI 10.1007/978-1-4939-0005-3_3,
© Springer Science+Business Media New York 2014

used in this chapter, the   —R— codes (R Development Core
Team, 2008) are provided in Appendix.

3.1   Quantile Function

Before defining the quantile residual life function, let us define the
quantile function first. When there is no censoring, suppose that
T is time to an event with the survival function $S(t) = \Pr(T > t)$.
The τ-quantile function under the survival function is generally
defined as $\theta_\tau \equiv S^{-1}(\tau) = \inf\{t : S(t) \leq \tau\}$, or $F^{-1}(\tau) = \inf\{t :
F(t) \geq \tau\}$ under the cumulative distribution function $F(\cdot)$ (see
Fig. 3.1). This Inversion Formula gives the median when $\tau = 1/2$.

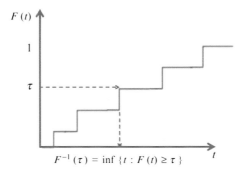

Fig. 3.1: The τ-quantile function

3.1.1   Asymptotic Variance Formula

Suppose $T_1, T_2, \ldots, T_n$ is a random sample from a continuous distribution with the probability density function $f(t)$, t_τ defines the
τ-quantile $(0 < \tau < 1)$, and $T_{(k)}$ is the kth order statistic. Since
the probability density function of $T_{(k)}$ is given by

$$g_k(t_{(k)}) = \frac{n!}{(k-1)!(n-k)!} F(t_{(k)})^{k-1}\{1 - F(t_{(k)})\}^{n-k} f(t_{(k)}),$$

$U_{(k)} \equiv F(T_{(k)})$ follows a Beta$(k, n - k + 1)$ distribution after the
change of variable, which has the mean $k/(n+1)$ and the variance

$$\frac{\{k/(n+1)\}\{1 - k/(n+1)\}}{n+2} \approx \frac{\tau(1-\tau)}{n},$$

as $n \to \infty$ and $k/n \to \tau$. By using the delta method, the asymptotic variance of the τ-quantile $T_{(k)} = F^{-1}(U_{(k)})$ is given by

$$\mathrm{Var}(T_{(k)}) = \mathrm{Var}(U_{(k)})(dt_{(k)}/du_{(k)})^2 = \{\tau(1-\tau)\}/nf(\theta_\tau)^2.$$

3.1.2 Asymptotic Normality

We will show the asymptotic normality of the quantile function by using the fact that the sample quantile function is a linear function of the influence functions (asymptotic linearity).

Let us first define the influence function. Suppose $T_1, T_2, \ldots, T_n$ is a random sample from a population with the cumulative distribution function F. The empirical distribution of F is defined as $F_n(t) = (1/n)\sum_{i=1}^{n} \Delta_{x_i}(t)$, where $\Delta_x(t)$ is the point mass 1 at x defined as an indicator function $I(t \geq x) = 1_{[x,\infty)}(t)$. Denote $\phi(F_n) = \phi_n(T_1, T_2, \ldots, T_n)$ as an estimator for the parameter of interest, and $\phi(F)$ as the limiting value of $\phi(F_n)$ as $n \to \infty$. For example, $\phi(F)$ and $\phi(F_n)$ can be the population mean with the distribution function F and the corresponding sample mean, respectively. The influence function is theoretically defined as

$$IF(x; \phi, F) = \lim_{\epsilon \to 0} \frac{\phi((1-\epsilon)F + \epsilon\Delta_x) - \phi(F)}{\epsilon},$$

but we start from the finite-sample version of Tukey's sensitivity curve (SC) (1977) for clearer interpretation of this function. The sample SC curve is defined as n times the change of $\phi(F_n)$ caused by an additional observation in x, i.e.

$$SC_n(x) = n[\phi_n(t_1, t_2, \ldots, t_{n-1}, x) - \phi_{n-1}(t_1, t_2, \ldots, t_{n-1})],$$

which, by translating and rescaling, can be rewritten as

$$SC_n(x) = \left[\phi\left(\left(1 - \frac{1}{n}\right)F_{n-1} + \frac{1}{n}\Delta_x\right) - \phi(F_{n-1})\right] / \left(\frac{1}{n}\right),$$

when $\phi_n(t_1, t_2, \ldots, t_n) = \phi(F_n)$ for any n, any sample $(t_1, t_2, \ldots, t_n)$, and corresponding empirical distribution F_n. Replacing $1/n$ and F_n with ϵ and F, respectively, gives the definition of the influence function in the above. Therefore the interpretation of the influence function would be the change in the value $\phi(F)$ if an infinitesimally small part of F is replaced by a point mass at x, which is also referred to as *Gâteaux derivative* (Gâteaux, 1913, 1919).

The asymptotic linearity plays an important role in establishing the asymptotic normality of the sampling distribution of a statistic.

Definiton 2.1 (Asymptotic Linearity). A statistic V_n is asymptotically linear $AL(\nu, k(\cdot), \tau^2)$ if there exists a finite and positive function of random variables $IF(\cdot)$ with $E[IF(T)] = 0$ and $\mathrm{var}[IF(T)] = \tau^2$ such that

$$V_n = \nu + \frac{1}{n}\sum_{i=1}^{n} IF(T_i) + o_p(1/\sqrt{n}),$$

where $IF(\cdot)$ is the influence function. As a simple example, the sample mean $\bar{T}_n$ is $AL(\mu, IF(\cdot), \sigma^2)$ with $IF(t) = t - \mu$, which has mean 0 and variance σ^2. Ignoring the error term, $IF(T_i)/n$ is the amount that T_i pulls V_n away from its limiting value ν. Since we are dealing with the quantile function, which is a function of the distribution function, i.e. $\phi(F) = F^{-1}(\tau)$, we need to find the influence function of $\phi(F)$

$$\left[\frac{d}{d\epsilon}\phi\left((1-\epsilon)F(t) + \epsilon\Delta_x(t)\right)\right]_{|\epsilon=0}.$$

Setting $F_\epsilon(t) = (1-\epsilon)F(t) + \epsilon\Delta_x(t)$ implies

$$\tau = F_\epsilon\left(F_\epsilon^{-1}(\tau)\right) = (1-\epsilon)F\left(F_\epsilon^{-1}(\tau)\right) + \epsilon\Delta_x\left(F_\epsilon^{-1}(\tau)\right).$$

By differentiating both sides with respect to ϵ, we have

$$0 = -F\left(F_\epsilon^{-1}(\tau)\right) + f\left(F_\epsilon^{-1}(\tau)\right)\left[\frac{d}{d\epsilon}F_\epsilon^{-1}(\tau)\right] + \Delta_x\left(F_\epsilon^{-1}(\tau)\right),$$

which gives the influence function of the quantile function at $\epsilon = 0$ as

$$\left[\frac{d}{d\epsilon}F_\epsilon^{-1}(\tau)\right]_{|\epsilon=0} = \left[\frac{d}{d\epsilon}\phi\left((1-\epsilon)F(t) + \epsilon\Delta_x(t)\right)\right]_{|\epsilon=0}$$

$$= -\frac{1_{[x,\infty)}\left(F^{-1}(\tau)\right) - \tau}{f\left(F^{-1}(\tau)\right)}.$$

Finally the Bahadur Representation Theorem (Bahadur, 1966) asserts that the sample quantiles are asymptotically linear because they can be expressed with the error term of order $o_p(1/\sqrt{n})$ as

$$F_n^{-1}(\tau) = F^{-1}(\tau) - \frac{1}{n} \sum_{i=1}^{n} \frac{1_{[x_i,\infty)}\left(F^{-1}(\tau)\right) - \tau}{f\left(F^{-1}(\tau)\right)} + o_p(1/\sqrt{n}), \quad (3.1)$$

which is equivalent to

$$\sqrt{n}\left[F_n^{-1}(\tau) - F^{-1}(\tau)\right] = -\frac{1}{\sqrt{n}} \sum_{i=1}^{n} \frac{1_{[x_i,\infty)}\left(F^{-1}(\tau)\right) - \tau}{f\left(F^{-1}(\tau)\right)} + o_p(1).$$

By the central limit theorem (CLT), we have the asymptotic normality (AN)

$$\sqrt{n}\left[F_n^{-1}(\tau) - F^{-1}(\tau)\right] \sim AN\left(0, \frac{\tau(1-\tau)}{f\left(F^{-1}(\tau)\right)^2}\right),$$

which also implies that the sample τ-quantile $F_n^{-1}(\tau)$ is an asymptotically consistent estimator of the population τ-quantile $F^{-1}(\tau)$ because $\lim_{n\to\infty} E[F_n^{-1}(\tau)] = F^{-1}(\tau)$. Shorack and Wellner (2009, p. 638) also show that the quantile process converges to a Brownian bridge.

3.2 Quantile Residual Life Function

We first consider the median residual life function, which is a special case of the quantile residual life function and has been popular in the literature. The median residual life function is defined as the median of the remaining lifetimes among survivors beyond time t_0, or more formally $\theta(t_0) = \text{median}(T_i - t_0 | T_i > t_0)$. In other words, half the population is below or above $\theta(t_0)$ under the distribution of the remaining lifetimes $T_i - t_0$ at a fixed time point t_0. Dropping the subscripts, this definition is equivalent to

Table 3.1: Survival functions and corresponding median residual life function (MDRL) for various distribution functions

Distribution	Survival function, $S(t)$	MDRL, $\theta(t)$
Exponential	$\exp(-\lambda t)$	$\ln(2)/\lambda$
Weibull	$\exp(-\lambda t^\kappa)$	$\{\ln(2)/\lambda + t^\kappa\}^{1/\kappa} - t$
Log-logistic	$(1 + \lambda t^\kappa)^{-1}$	$\lambda^{-1/\kappa}\{2(1 + \lambda t^\kappa) - 1\}^{1/\kappa} - t$
Pareto	$(1 + \lambda t)^{-\kappa}$	$(2^{1/\kappa} - 1)(t + 1/\lambda)$
Exponential power	$\exp[1 - \exp\{(\lambda t)^\kappa\}]$	$(1/\lambda)[\ln\{\ln(2) + \exp\{(\lambda t)^\kappa\}\}]^{1/\kappa} - t$

$$\Pr(T - t > \theta(t)|T > t) = 1/2, \tag{3.2}$$

which can be rewritten as $S(t + \theta(t)) = (1/2)S(t)$. Therefore for a continuous and strictly decreasing $S(t)$ with a closed form, the median residual lifetime $\theta(t)$ can be uniquely determined as

$$\theta(t) = S^{-1}[(1/2)S(t)] - t. \tag{3.3}$$

Table 3.1 summarizes the survival function and corresponding median residual life function for various distributions.

Example 3.1 (Exponential and Weibull). For the exponential distribution, because $S^{-1}(u) = -(1/\lambda)\ln(u)$, $\theta(t) = S^{-1}\left(\frac{1}{2}e^{-\lambda t}\right) - t = \ln(2)/\lambda$. In this case, note that the median residual life function is constant over time, which may not be suitable in practice. Figure 3.2 plots the pattern of the median residual life for the Weibull distribution with the scale parameter $\lambda = 0.05$ and different values of the shape parameter κ over the time window between 0 and 10. One can observe that $\theta(t)$ increases and decreases over time when $\kappa < 1$ and $\kappa > 1$, respectively.

In general, the τ-quantile residual life function is defined as $\theta^{(\tau)}(t) = \tau\text{-percentile}(T - t|T > t)$, so that

$$\Pr(T - t > \theta^{(\tau)}(t)|T > t) = 1 - \tau. \tag{3.4}$$

The quantile residual life function enjoys the following properties (Bandos, 2007):

1. $\theta^{(\tau)}(t) \geq 0$ and $\theta^{(\tau)}(0) = \text{quantile}(T)$

2. $\theta^{(\tau)}(t) + t = S^{-1}\left[(1-\tau)S(t)\right]$ is always nondecreasing

3. The median residual life function does not uniquely define the underlying distribution while the mean residual life function does (Joe and Proschan, 1984; Gupta and Langford, 1984)

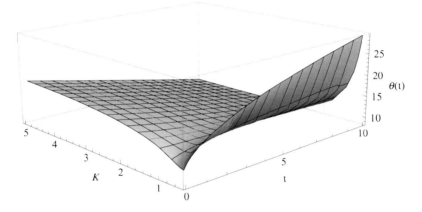

Fig. 3.2: A graph of the median residual life function from Weibull distribution

3.3 Quantile Residual Life Process

As defined in Sect. 3.2, the τ-quantile residual life function at a time point t is defined as

$$\theta^{(\tau)}(t) = S^{-1}\left[(1-\tau)S(t)\right] - t. \tag{3.5}$$

Without censoring, the survival function $S(\cdot)$ can be estimated by the complement of the empirical cumulative distribution function estimate, i.e. $S_n(\cdot) = 1 - F_n(\cdot)$, which can be inverted by $S_n^{-1}(u) = \inf\{t : S_n(t) \leq u\}$. When there is censoring, the Kaplan–Meier estimator (Kaplan and Meier, 1958) would be a reasonable choice to replace $S_n(\cdot)$. Figure 3.3 shows graphically how the median residual life function can be nonparametrically estimated.

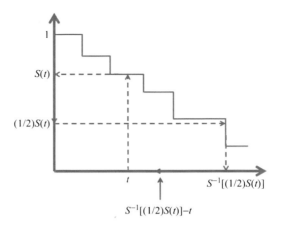

Fig. 3.3: Graphical presentation of how the median residual life can be estimated by inverting the estimated survival function

Following Shorack and Wellner (2009), we show here that the sample quantile residual life process converges to a Brown bridge. Let us consider a process of $Q_n(t) = \sqrt{n}\left[\theta_n^{(\tau)}(t) - \theta^{(\tau)}(t)\right]$ where

$$\theta_n^{(\tau)}(t) = S_n^{-1}\left[(1-\tau)S_n(t)\right] - t$$

is the sample quantile residual life process. By defining $\xi_n(t) = (1-\tau)S_n(t)$ with its limiting value of $\xi(t)$, we have

$$
\begin{aligned}
Q_n(t) &= \sqrt{n}\left[S_n^{-1}(\xi_n(t)) - S^{-1}(\xi(t))\right] \\
&= \sqrt{n}\left[S^{-1}\left\{S(S_n^{-1}(\xi_n(t)))\right\} - S^{-1}(\xi(t))\right] \\
&= \frac{S^{-1}\left\{S(S_n^{-1}(\xi_n(t)))\right\} - S^{-1}(\xi(t))}{S(S_n^{-1}(\xi_n(t))) - \xi(t)} \\
&\quad \times \sqrt{n}\left[S(S_n^{-1}(\xi_n(t))) - \xi(t)\right].
\end{aligned}
\tag{3.6}
$$

Note that ξ_{ni} $(i = 1,\ldots,n)$ is a random sample from the uniform distribution $(0,1)$ for a fixed value of τ and $S(S_n^{-1}(\xi_n(t)))$ is equivalent to the quantile process of the ordered uniform random variables, $\xi_{n:1},\ldots,\xi_{n:n}$, i.e. $S(S_n^{-1}(\xi_n(t))) \equiv G_n^{-1}(\xi_n(t))$, where G_n is the empirical distribution function of ξ_{ni}'s, if the true survival function intersects the vertical line of the empirical survival function at $S_n^{-1}(\xi_n(t))$ (Fig. 3.4). This would occur almost surely by the Glivenko–Cantelli theorem as $n \to \infty$ (see also Csörgő (1983)). Here note that the vertical lines of the empirical survival function are the quantile function of the uniform random variables, ξ_{ni}'s $(i = 1, \ldots, n)$.

Therefore, defining

$$A_n = \frac{S^{-1}\left[G_n^{-1}(\xi_n(t))\right] - S^{-1}(\xi(t))}{G_n^{-1}(\xi_n(t)) - \xi(t)},$$

Eq. (3.6) is now equivalent to

$$
\begin{aligned}
Q_n(t) &= A_n \sqrt{n}\left[G_n^{-1}(\xi_n(t)) - \xi(t)\right] \\
&= A_n \sqrt{n}\left[G_n^{-1}(\xi_n(t)) - \xi_n(t) - \{\xi(t) - \xi_n(t)\}\right] \\
&= A_n \sqrt{n}\left[G_n^{-1}(\xi_n(t)) - \xi_n(t) - (1-\tau)\{S(t) - S_n(t)\}\right].
\end{aligned}
$$

As $n \to \infty$, the uniform quantile process $\sqrt{n}[G_n^{-1}(\xi_n(t)) - \xi_n(t)]$ converges to a Brownian bridge $-B(\xi(t))$ (Shorack and Wellner, 2009, p. 86), the empirical process of the survival function $\sqrt{n}[S(t) - S_n(t)] = -\sqrt{n}[S_n(t) - S(t)]$ converges to a Brownian bridge $-B(S(t))$, and we have

$$
\begin{aligned}
\lim_{n\to\infty} A_n &= \lim_{n\to\infty} \frac{S^{-1}\left[G_n^{-1}(\xi_n(t))\right] - S^{-1}(\xi(t))}{G_n^{-1}(\xi_n(t)) - \xi(t)} \\
&= \frac{dS^{-1}(\xi(t))}{d\xi(t)} = -\frac{1}{f(\xi(t))},
\end{aligned}
$$

since $\sup|G_n^{-1}(\xi_n(t) - \xi(t)| \to 0$ a.s. as $n \to \infty$ by the Glivenko–Cantelli theorem (Shorack and Wellner, 2009, p. 95). Putting all these together, we have just shown that the quantile residual life process $f(\xi(t))Q_n(t)$ converges to a Brownian bridge

$$B((1-\tau)S(t)) - (1-\tau)B(S(t)).$$

The variance of the Brownian bridge is given by $\mathrm{Var}\{B((1-\tau)S(t))\} + (1-\tau)^2\mathrm{Var}\{B(S(t)\} - 2(1-\tau)\mathrm{Cov}\{B(1-\tau)S(t)), B(S(t))\} = (1-\tau)S(t)\{1 - (1-\tau)S(t)\} + (1-\tau)^2 S(t)\{1 - S(t)\} - 2(1-\tau)\{(1-\tau)S(t) - (1-\tau)S(t)^2\} = (1-\tau)S(t)$, since $S(t) > \tau(1-\tau)S(t)$, which coincides with the results in Csörgő and Csörgő (1987).

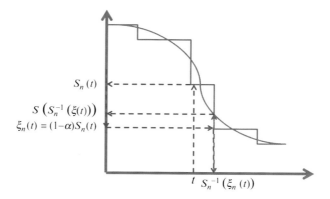

Fig. 3.4: Graphical presentation of equivalence of $S(S_n^{-1}(\xi_n(t)))$ and $G_n^{-1}(\xi_n(t))$

3.4   Parametric Inference

Parametric methods would provide more accurate inference results if the data fit the assumed distribution or model reasonably well. In this section, we outline the maximum likelihood principle to infer the quantile residual life function for one-sample case and a difference between two quantile residual lifetimes. One major advantage of the parametric approach would be that estimation of the probability density function to evaluate the variance of the quantile estimator does not need a smoothing technique.

3.4.1   One-Sample Case

From the definition of the τ-quantile residual life function given in (3.4), the cumulative distribution function of the residual life distribution at time $t = t_0$, denoted by $F_{t_0}(t)$, can be defined in terms of the cumulative distribution function $F(t)$ and survival function $S(t)$ at the origin as follows:

$$F_{t_0}(t; \boldsymbol{\psi}) = \frac{F(t + t_0; \boldsymbol{\psi}) - F(t_0; \boldsymbol{\psi})}{S(t_0; \boldsymbol{\psi})}, \tag{3.7}$$

where $\boldsymbol{\psi}$ is a vector of parameters. By setting Eq. (3.7) equal to τ and solving it for t gives the τ-quantile residual life function, $\theta_{t_0}(\tau; \boldsymbol{\psi})$, as

$$\theta_{t_0}(\tau; \boldsymbol{\psi}) = F^{-1}[F(t_0; \boldsymbol{\psi}) + \tau S(t_0; \boldsymbol{\psi})] - t_0, \qquad (3.8)$$

which is a function of the parameters for the distribution at the origin, once a closed form of the distribution function is provided as in Table 3.1. Therefore, parametric inference on the τ-quantile residual life function would be straightforward by using the invariance property of the maximum likelihood estimator. We consider the right censoring here, which would include an uncensored case as a special case. For the ith subject, define T_i as the potential event time and C_i as the potential censoring time, so that we observe the minimum, i.e. $X_i = \min(T_i, C_i)$. Then an event indicator function is $\delta_i = I(T_i \le C_i)$. Based on the observable random variable (X_i, δ_i) and under the independence assumption between T_i and C_i, the maximum likelihood function is given by

$$
\begin{aligned}
L(\boldsymbol{\psi}; x_i, \delta_i) &= \prod_{i=1}^{n} f(\boldsymbol{\psi}; x_i)^{\delta_i} S(\boldsymbol{\psi}; x_i)^{1-\delta_i} \\
&= \prod_{i=1}^{n} h(\boldsymbol{\psi}; x_i)^{\delta_i} S(\boldsymbol{\psi}; x_i),
\end{aligned}
$$

where $f(x) = -dS(x)/dx$ and $h(x) = f(x)/S(x)$ are the probability density function and hazard function of T, respectively. The maximum likelihood estimate(s) (MLE) of $\boldsymbol{\psi}$ can be obtained by taking the first derivative of the logarithm of the likelihood function, setting it to 0, and solve the equation simultaneously for the parameters in $\boldsymbol{\psi}$. Let us denote the MLE as $\hat{\boldsymbol{\psi}}$, which will be asymptotically consistent and normally distributed. By plugging the consistent estimator $\hat{\boldsymbol{\psi}}$ into (3.7), the cumulative distribution function of the residual life distribution can be consistently estimated as $F_{t_0}(x; \hat{\boldsymbol{\psi}})$ with its asymptotic variance

$$\text{Var}\left[F_{t_0}(x; \hat{\boldsymbol{\psi}})\right] = \left(\frac{\partial F_{t_0}(x; \boldsymbol{\psi})}{\partial \boldsymbol{\psi}}\right)^T I^{-1}(\boldsymbol{\psi}) \left(\frac{\partial F_{t_0}(x; \boldsymbol{\psi})}{\partial \boldsymbol{\psi}}\right),$$

where $\partial F_{t_0}(x; \boldsymbol{\psi})/\partial \boldsymbol{\psi}$ is a vector containing the first derivatives of the residual life distribution function $F_{t_0}(x; \boldsymbol{\psi})$ with respect to the parameter vector $\boldsymbol{\psi}$, and $I(\boldsymbol{\psi})$ is the Fisher information matrix, i.e. the expectation of the negative second derivatives of the log-likelihood function with respect to the parameter vector $\boldsymbol{\psi}$. The Fisher information matrix is often replaced by the observed information matrix in practice.

Because the quantile residual life function $\theta_{t_0}(\tau; \boldsymbol{\psi})$ is the inverse transformation of the residual life cumulative distribution function $F_{t_0}(t; \boldsymbol{\psi})$ and hence a function of $\boldsymbol{\psi}$, application of the delta method gives

$$\text{Var}\left[\theta_{t_0}(\tau; \hat{\boldsymbol{\psi}})\right] = (1/f_{t_0}(\theta_{t_0}(\tau; \boldsymbol{\psi}); \boldsymbol{\psi}))^2 \text{Var}\left[F_{t_0}(\theta_{t_0}(\tau; \boldsymbol{\psi}); \hat{\boldsymbol{\psi}})\right],$$

(3.9)

where

$$\theta_{t_0}(\tau; \hat{\boldsymbol{\psi}}) = F^{-1}[F(t_0; \hat{\boldsymbol{\psi}}) + \tau S(t_0; \hat{\boldsymbol{\psi}})] - t_0$$

and

$$f_{t_0}(t; \boldsymbol{\psi}) = \frac{\partial F_{t_0}(t; \boldsymbol{\psi})}{\partial t} = \frac{f(t + t_0; \boldsymbol{\psi})}{S(t_0; \boldsymbol{\psi})}.$$

(3.10)

The asymptotic variance of $\theta_{t_0}(\tau; \hat{\boldsymbol{\psi}})$ can be consistently estimated by replacing $\boldsymbol{\psi}$, $\theta_{t_0}(\tau; \boldsymbol{\psi})$, and $f_{t_0}(\theta_{t_0}(\tau; \boldsymbol{\psi}); \boldsymbol{\psi})$ with the maximum likelihood estimates $\hat{\boldsymbol{\psi}}$, $\theta_{t_0}(\tau; \hat{\boldsymbol{\psi}})$, and $f_{t_0}(\theta_{t_0}(\tau; \hat{\boldsymbol{\psi}}); \hat{\boldsymbol{\psi}})$.

Example 3.2 (Exponential Distribution with Censoring). For simplicity, let us consider the exponential distribution with a rate parameter λ, so that $S(t; \lambda) = \exp(-\lambda t)$. The log-likelihood function is given by

$$l \equiv \ln L(\lambda; x_i, \delta_i) = \sum_{i=1}^{n} \{\delta_i \ln(\lambda) - \lambda x_i\}.$$

Taking the first derivative of l with respect to λ and setting it to 0 gives the ML estimating equation

$$(1/\lambda)\left\{\sum_{i=1}^{n}(\delta_i - \lambda x_i)\right\} = 0,$$

which yields the MLE for λ as

$$\hat{\lambda} = \sum_{i=1}^{n}\delta_i / \sum_{i=1}^{n}x_i.$$

To find the variance of $\hat{\lambda}$, the negative second derivative of the log-likelihood function is given by $\sum_{i=1}^{n} \delta_i/\lambda^2$, which can be actually estimated from the data to be an observed information. The Fisher information can be obtained by taking expectation of the observed information as

$$
\begin{aligned}
I(\lambda) &= (n/\lambda^2)E(\delta_i) \\
&= (n/\lambda^2)E[E\{I(T \leq C)|T = t\}] \\
&= (n/\lambda^2)E\{\Pr(T \leq C|T = t)\} \\
&= (n/\lambda^2)E\{\Pr(C \geq t|T = t)\},
\end{aligned}
$$

which reduces to

$$
-(n/\lambda^2) \int_0^\infty G(v; \eta) dS(v; \lambda)
$$

when T and C are independent, where $G(v; \eta)$ is a parametric form of the survival function for C. Finally the variance of $\hat{\lambda}$ is given by

$$
\mathrm{Var}(\hat{\lambda}) = I^{-1}(\lambda) = \frac{\lambda^2}{-n \int_0^\infty G(v; \eta) dS(v; \lambda)},
$$

which is estimable once the data are observed. Note that when there is no censoring the variance formula reduces to λ^2/n because $\Pr(T \leq C) = 1$, implying that censoring would inflate the variance of the estimator $\hat{\lambda}$.

Now, from Table 3.1, the MLE for the median residual life function for the exponential distribution is given by $\theta_{t_0}(1/2; \hat{\lambda}) = \ln(2)/\hat{\lambda}$. To obtain the variance of $\theta_{t_0}(1/2; \hat{\lambda})$, we note that $F_{t_0}(t; \lambda) = 1 - \exp(-\lambda t)$ from (3.10) and hence $\partial F_{t_0}(t; \lambda)/\partial \lambda = t \exp(-\lambda t)$, which gives

$$
\mathrm{Var}\left[F_{t_0}(t; \hat{\lambda})\right] = \{t \exp(-\lambda t)\}^2 I^{-1}(\lambda).
$$

Finally, since $\partial F_{t_0}(t; \lambda)/\partial t = f_{t_0}(t; \lambda) = \lambda \exp(-\lambda t)$, the formula (3.9) gives

$$
\mathrm{Var}\left[\theta_{t_0}(1/2; \hat{\lambda})\right] = \frac{\{\ln(2)\}^2}{-n\lambda^2 \int_0^\infty G(v; \eta) dS(v; \lambda)},
$$

which can be consistently estimated by

$$\widehat{\text{Var}} \left[\theta_{t_0}(1/2; \hat{\lambda}) \right] \frac{\{\ln(2)\}^2}{-n\hat{\lambda}^2 \int_0^\infty G(v; \hat{\eta})dS(v; \hat{\lambda})},$$

where $G(v; \hat{\eta})$ and $S(v; \hat{\lambda})$ are the parametric estimates of the survival functions of T and C.

When the distribution under consideration involves more than one parameters such as in Weibull distribution, it is common that no closed form of the MLE exists, so that a numerical method such as the Newton–Raphson (Cajori, 1911) needs to be used to maximize the log-likelihood function.

3.4.2   Independent Two-Sample Case

Investigators would often be interested in comparing two quantile residual lifetimes to evaluate, say, a therapeutic effect of a new drug. For example, suppose a patient is being followed after the initial treatment for a disease, and in the middle of the follow-up period, a new drug is developed to prevent or delay a relapse of the disease. To assess this new drug for a secondary therapy, a study can be designed to compare the median residual lifetimes to a relapse between patients with or without the secondary therapy.

The results obtained for one-sample case presented in the previous section can be directly extended to a two-sample case by using the nice asymptotic properties of the maximum likelihood estimators. Suppose $\theta_{t_0}^{(k)}(\tau; \psi^{(k)})$ denote the τ-quantile from a residual life distribution for group k $(k = 1, 2)$ at time t_0. Because the estimator $\theta_{t_0}^{(k)}(\tau; \hat{\psi}^{(k)})$ asymptotically follows the normal distribution with mean $\theta_{t_0}^{(k)}(\tau; \psi^{(k)})$ and the variance given in (3.9) for each group k, under the null hypothesis of $H_0 : \theta_{t_0}^{(1)}(\tau; \psi^{(1)}) = \theta_{t_0}^{(2)}(\tau; \psi^{(2)})$, a two-sample statistic can be constructed as

$$W_{t_0}(\tau) = \frac{\theta_{t_0}^{(1)}(\tau; \hat{\psi}^{(1)}) - \theta_{t_0}^{(2)}(\tau; \hat{\psi}^{(2)})}{\sqrt{\widehat{\text{Var}} \left[\theta_{t_0}(\tau; \hat{\psi}^{(pooled)}) \right] + \widehat{\text{Var}} \left[\theta_{t_0}(\tau; \hat{\psi}^{(pooled)}) \right]}},$$

$$\tag{3.11}$$

where $\theta_{t_0}(\tau; \hat{\psi}^{(pooled)})$ is the τ-quantile residual life estimates from the pooled sample. The statistic (3.11) would converge in distribution to the standard normal distribution with mean 0 and variance 1 by the Slutsky's theorem (Slutsky, 1925). Here $\widehat{\text{Var}}\left[\theta_{t_0}(\tau; \hat{\psi}^{(pooled)})\right]$ is the consistent estimator for the variance of $\theta_{t_0}(\tau; \hat{\psi}^{(pooled)})$. For a two-sided test, a small or large value of $W_{t_0}(\tau)$ would reject the null hypothesis given a significance level.

3.5 Nonparametric Inference

First we begin with a brief literature review in nonparametric analysis of the quantile or the quantile residual life. Wang and Hettmansperger (1990) proposed a confidence interval approach to compare two quantiles from failure time distributions, but not for the residual life distributions. Since their method involves estimation of the probability density function under censoring, Su and Wei (1993) introduced a nonparametric test statistic by using the minimum dispersion statistic (Basawa and Koul, 1988). To generalize the previous results to a residual life distribution, Berger, Boos, and Guess (1988) proposed a modified test statistic based on Fligner and Rust's approach (1982) to compare two median *residual* lifetimes, which also required estimation of the probability density function. To overcome this disadvantage, Jeong, Jung, and Costantino (2007) extended Su and Wei's method to compare median residual lifetimes based on the minimum dispersion statistic. Here we elaborate on the two-sample statistic for the median residual life proposed by Jeong *et al.* (2007), but the results can be easily generalized to the τ-quantile.

3.5.1 One-Sample Case

Let us define T_i and C_i $(i = 1, 2, \ldots, n)$ as potential failure time and censoring time, respectively, and assume that they are independent. For the ith subject, let us denote $X_i = \min(T_i, C_i)$ for an observed survival time and $\delta_i = I(T_i \leq C_i)$ for an associated indicator function. For one-sample case, the survivor function of the residual lifetime for a patient who has survived beyond time

t_0, i.e. $(T_i - t_0 | T_i > t_0)$, is given as $S(t|t_0) = S(t + t_0)/S(t_0)$ for $t_0 \geq 0$. Denoting θ_{t_0} for the true median residual lifetime at t_0, it would be natural to estimate θ_{t_0} by solving the following equation for θ_{t_0}:

$$u(\theta_{t_0}) = \hat{S}(t_0 + \theta_{t_0}) - \frac{1}{2}\hat{S}(t_0) = 0, \qquad (3.12)$$

where $\hat{S}(t)$ is the Kaplan–Meier estimator of $S(t)$ based on (X_i, δ_i) $(i = 1, 2, \ldots, n)$. Equation (3.12) can be written in general for the τ-quantile as

$$u(\theta_{t_0}) = \hat{S}(t_0 + \theta_{t_0}) - (1 - \tau)\hat{S}(t_0) = 0.$$

Let's define the median residual life estimator from (3.12) as

$$\hat{\theta}_{t_0} = \hat{S}^{-1}((1/2)\hat{S}(t_0)) - t_0,$$

which can be heuristically shown to be the consistent estimator of θ_{t_0}. First, Fleming and Harrington (1991, Theorem 3.4.2) proved that the Kaplan–Meier estimator $\hat{S}(t)$ is uniformly consistent with the true curve $S(t)$ over $0 \leq t \leq M$, where $M = \sup\{t : \Pr(X > t) > 0\}$. Hence, for $t_0 + \theta_{t_0} < M$, $u(\theta_{t_0})$ uniformly converges to

$$\dot{u}(\theta_{t_0}) = S(t_0 + \theta_{t_0}) - \frac{1}{2}S(t_0). \qquad (3.13)$$

Recalling that θ_{t_0} denotes for the true value of the median residual lifetime at time t_0, we have $\dot{u}(\theta_{t_0}) = 0$, and consequently $\hat{\theta}_{t_0}$ is a consistent estimator of θ_{t_0}.

Once data are observed, it would be straightforward to obtain the median residual life estimate $\hat{\theta}_{t_0}$. As shown in Sect. 3.3, however, the variance of the quantile residual life estimator would involve the probability density function of the underlying true failure time distribution under censoring. Therefore, to infer the true median residual life function, we adopt to construct a test statistic based on the entire estimating function (3.12) via the martingale representation of the Kaplan–Meier estimator. For a large sample from a continuous true survival function $S(t)$, from Eq. (1.7) in Sect. 1.5.4 the Kaplan–Meier process $\hat{S}(t) - S(t)$ can be expressed as a martingale

$$\hat{S}(t) - S(t) = -S(t) \int_0^t \frac{dM(v)}{Y(v)} + o_p(n^{-1/2}), \qquad (3.14)$$

where $M(t) = \sum_{i=1}^{n} M_i(t) = \sum_{i=1}^{n} N_i(t) - \sum_{i=1}^{n} \int_0^t Y_i(v)dH(v)$ is the basic counting process martingale defined in Sect. 1.5.3. Therefore the process (3.14) can be re-expressed as

$$\hat{S}(t) - S(t) = -S(t) \sum_{i=1}^{n} \int_0^t \frac{dM_i(v)}{Y(v)} + o_p(n^{-1/2}), \qquad (3.15)$$

where $M_i(t) = N_i(t) - \int_0^t Y_i(v)dH(v)$ is an individual martingale. Here $o_p(n^{-1/2})$ implies that the remainder terms converge in probability to 0 after being multiplied by $\sqrt{n}$. By using this martingale representation of the Kaplan–Meier process in (3.15), the estimating equation in (3.12) can be expressed as

$$
\begin{aligned}
u(\theta_{t_0}) = \ & -S(t_0 + \theta_{t_0}) \sum_{i=1}^{n} \int_0^{t_0+\theta_{t_0}} \frac{dM_i(v)}{Y(v)} + S(t_0 + \theta_{t_0}) \\
& -\frac{1}{2}\left\{ -S(t_0) \sum_{i=1}^{n} \int_0^{t_0} \frac{dM_i(v)}{Y(v)} + S(t_0) \right\} + o_p(n^{-1/2}),
\end{aligned}
$$

which reduces to

$$
\begin{aligned}
u(\theta_{t_0}) = \ & -S(t_0 + \theta_{t_0}) \sum_{i=1}^{n} \int_0^{t_0+\theta_{t_0}} \frac{dM_i(v)}{Y(v)} \\
& +\frac{1}{2}S(t_0) \sum_{i=1}^{n} \int_0^{t_0} \frac{dM_i(v)}{Y(v)} + o_p(n^{-1/2}),
\end{aligned}
$$

because $\dot{u}(\theta_{t_0}) = 0$ from (3.13).

After replacing $Y(t)/n$ with its limiting value $y(t)$, we obtain

$$u(\theta_{t_0}) = \sum_{i=1}^{n} e_i(\theta_{t_0}) + o_p(n^{-1/2}),$$

where

$$e_i(x) = -S(t_0 + x) \int_0^{t_0+x} \frac{dM_i(v)}{ny(v)} + \frac{1}{2}S(t_0) \int_0^{t_0} \frac{dM_i(v)}{ny(v)} \qquad (3.16)$$

are independent random variables with mean 0 because

$$E\{dM_i(t)\} = E[E\{dM_i(t)|\mathcal{F}_t\}] = 0$$

for a filtration $\{\mathcal{F}_t : t \geq 0\}$. Again because $\dot{u}(\theta_{t_0}) = 0$ from (3.13), which implies $S(t_0 + \theta_{t_0}) = (1/2)S(t_0)$, Eq. (3.16) further simplifies to

$$e_i(x) = -\frac{1}{2}S(t_0)\int_{t_0}^{t_0+x}\frac{dM_i(v)}{ny(v)}.$$

The CLT justifies that $u(\theta_{t_0})$ would follow an asymptotically normal distribution with mean 0 and variance $\sigma_{t_0}^2(\theta_{t_0}) = \sum_{i=1}^{n} e_i^2(\theta_{t_0})$ assuming that $e_i(\theta_{t_0})$'s are identically distributed.

The variance can be simply estimated by replacing $e_i(\theta_{t_0,0})$ with its consistent estimate $\hat{e}_i(\hat{\theta}_{t_0})$, where

$$\hat{e}_i(x) = -\frac{1}{2}\hat{S}(t_0)\int_{t_0}^{t_0+x}\frac{d\hat{M}_i(v)}{Y(v)}, \tag{3.17}$$

and $\hat{M}_i(t) = N_i(t) - \int_0^t Y_i(v)d\hat{H}(v)$ and $\hat{H}(t) = \int_0^t Y^{-1}(v)dN(v)$ is the Nelson-Aalen estimator (Nelson, 1972; Aalen, 1975) of the cumulative hazard function.

To test the null hypothesis of $H_0 : \theta_{t_0} = m_0$, one-sample test statistic can be constructed as

$$V(m_0) = \frac{\hat{u}^2(m_0)}{\hat{\sigma}_{t_0}^2(\hat{\theta}_{t_0})}, \tag{3.18}$$

where $\hat{u}(m_0) = \sum_{i=1}^{n} \hat{e}_i(m_0)$ and $\hat{\sigma}_{t_0}^2(\hat{\theta}_{t_0}) = \sum_{i=1}^{n} \hat{e}_i^2(\hat{\theta}_{t_0})$.

Since the Wald type statistic $\hat{u}(m_0)/\hat{\sigma}_{t_0}(\hat{\theta}_{t_0})$ follows asymptotically the standard normal distribution under the null hypothesis by the Slutsky's theorem, the test statistic (3.18) would follow a χ^2-distribution with 1 degree of freedom, so that a large value of $V(m_0)$ would reject the null hypothesis. A $100 \times (1 - \alpha)\%$ confidence interval for θ_{t_0} can also be obtained from

$$\{\theta_{t_0} : \hat{u}(\theta_{t_0})^2/\hat{\sigma}_{t_0}^2(\hat{\theta}_{t_0}) < \chi_{1-\alpha,1}^2\}, \tag{3.19}$$

where $\chi_{1-\alpha,1}^2$ is the $100 \times (1-\alpha)^{th}$ percentile of the χ^2-distribution with 1 degree of freedom.

Example 3.3 (Numerical Calculation of One-Sample Test Statistic). In this example, we demonstrate numerical evaluation of the one-sample test statistic. First we simulate a dataset from a Weibull distribution with the survival function $S(t) = \exp(-\lambda t^\kappa)$, under which the true median residual life function at time t_0 is defined as (Table 3.1)

$$q_{t_0} = \{\ln(2)/\lambda + t_0^\kappa\}^{1/\kappa} - t_0. \qquad (3.20)$$

By using the probability integral transformation, the potential event time T_i can be generated from

$$T_i = \{-\log(1 - U_i)/\lambda\}^{1/\kappa},$$

where U_i is a random number from a Uniform distribution between 0 and 1. The potential censoring time C_i can be generated from a Uniform distribution between a and b, where a and b control the censoring proportion. Finally the observed survival time can be determined as the minimum of the potential event and censoring times, i.e. $X_i = \min(T_i, C_i)$. In this example, we have generated 10 observed survival times with associated event indicators after setting $\lambda = 0.09$, $\kappa = 2$, $a = 1.5$, and $b = 10$. Table 3.2 shows the observed survival times and event indicators. Figure 3.5 shows the Kaplan–Meier estimates based on this dataset.

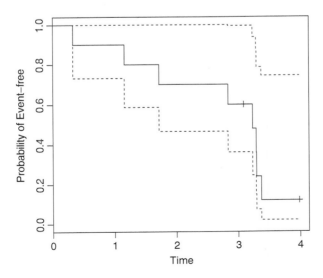

Fig. 3.5: Kaplan–Meier estimates for the simulated dataset

Table 3.2: A simulated dataset from a Weibull distribution: x_i, observed survival times; $\delta_i=1$ for event and 0 for censored

x_i, observed survival time	δ_i, event indicator
1.1580810	1
3.2891294	1
3.2313578	1
3.2939626	1
3.9846846	0
3.3706485	1
0.3255957	1
1.7149105	1
3.0871437	0
2.8324774	1

Since $(1/2)\hat{S}(t_0)$ and $\hat{S}(t_0+\theta_{t_0})$ may not be close to each other in practice, especially for a small sample, we will use a sample version of the formula (3.16). Denoting that $x_{(i)}$ $(i = 1, \ldots, n)$ is the ordered observed survival times (censored or uncensored), a sample version of the formula (3.16) at $\hat{\theta}_{t_0}$ can be written as

$$\hat{e}_i(\hat{\theta}_{t_0}) = -\hat{S}(t_0+\hat{\theta}_{t_0}) \int_0^{t_0+\hat{\theta}_{t_0}} \frac{d\hat{M}_i(v)}{Y(v)} + \frac{1}{2}\hat{S}(t_0) \int_0^{t_0} \frac{d\hat{M}_i(v)}{Y(v)}. \quad (3.21)$$

Since

$$d\hat{M}_i(v) = dN_i(v) - \frac{Y_i(v)dN(v)}{Y(v)},$$

the term

$$\int_0^{t_0+\hat{\theta}_{t_0}} \frac{d\hat{M}_i(v)}{Y(v)}$$

can be written in a discrete form as

$$\begin{aligned}
D_{i1} &= I_{[0,t_0+\hat{\theta}_{t_0}]}(x_{(i)}) \frac{dN_i(x_{(i)})}{Y(x_{(i)})} \\
&\quad - \sum_{j=1}^n I_{[0,\min(x_{(i)},t_0+\hat{\theta}_{t_0})]}(x_{(j)}) \frac{dN(x_{(j)})}{Y(x_{(j)})^2} \\
&\equiv D_{i1,1} - D_{i1,2}
\end{aligned}$$

where $I_{[a,b]}(t) = 1$ if $t \in [a,b]$ and 0 otherwise. Note that the first term of D_{i1}, $D_{i1,1}$, contributes by $1/Y(x_{(i)})$ only when $x_{(i)}$ is an event that occurs between 0 and $t_0 + \hat{\theta}_{t_0}$. The second term of D_{i1}, $D_{i1,2}$, contributes by the cumulative sum of $1/Y(x_{(i)})^2$ between 0 and $x_{(i)}$ if $x_{(i)}$ is between 0 and $t_0 + \hat{\theta}_{t_0}$ and by the cumulative sum of $1/Y(x_{(i)})^2$ between 0 and $t_0 + \hat{\theta}_{t_0}$ if $x_{(i)}$ is beyond $t_0 + \hat{\theta}_{t_0}$. Similarly the term

$$\int_0^{t_0} \frac{d\hat{M}_i(v)}{Y(v)}$$

can be written as

$$D_{i2} = I_{[0,t_0]}(x_{(i)}) \frac{dN_i(x_{(i)})}{Y(x_{(i)})} - \sum_{j=1}^{n} I_{[0,\min(x_{(i)},t_0)]}(x_{(j)}) \frac{dN(x_{(j)})}{Y(x_{(j)})^2}$$

$$\equiv D_{i2,1} - D_{i2,2},$$

so that we have

$$\hat{e}_i(\hat{\theta}_{t_0}) = -\hat{S}(t_0 + \hat{\theta}_{t_0}) D_{i1} + \frac{1}{2}\hat{S}(t_0) D_{i2}, \qquad (3.22)$$

where $\hat{S}(\cdot)$ is the Kaplan–Meier estimates.

Suppose that we are interested in evaluating one-sample statistic to infer the median residual lifetime at $t_0 = 2$. From Fig. 3.5 and Table 3.2, $\hat{S}(t_0) = 0.7$, so that the median residual life estimate is $\hat{\theta}_{t_0} = 1.294$ and $\hat{S}(t_0 + \hat{\theta}_{t_0}) = 0.24$. Table 3.3 shows the quantities needed to calculate $\hat{e}_i(\hat{\theta}_{t_0})$. For example for ID=9, we have

$$
\begin{aligned}
D_{i1,1} &= 0 \\
D_{i1,2} &= 1/10^2 + 1/9^2 + 1/8^2 + 1/7^2 + 1/5^2 + 1/4^2 + 1/3^2 = 0.272 \\
D_{i2,1} &= 0 \\
D_{i2,2} &= 1/10^2 + 1/9^2 + 1/8^2 = 0.038,
\end{aligned}
$$

which gives

$$
\begin{aligned}
\hat{e}_9(\hat{\theta}_{t_0}) &= -\hat{S}(t_0 + \hat{\theta}_{t_0}) D_{i1} + \frac{1}{2}\hat{S}(t_0) D_{i2} \\
&= -\hat{S}(3.294)(0 - 0.272) + \frac{1}{2}\hat{S}(2)(0 - 0.038) \\
&= -0.24 \times (-0.272) + 0.5 \times 0.70 \times (-0.038) = 0.052.
\end{aligned}
$$

Table 3.3: Quantities required for calculating $\hat{e}_i(\hat{\theta}_{t_0})$: $x_{(i)}$, ordered observed survival times; $dN(x_{(i)})$, increment of #events at $x_{(i)}$; $Y(x_{(i)})$, # of subjects at risk at $x_{(i)}$; $\hat{S}(x_{(i)})$, the Kaplan–Meier estimates; $I_1 = I_{[0,t_0]}(x_{(i)})$; $I_2 = I_{[0,t_0+\hat{\theta}_{t_0}]}(x_{(i)})$

ID	$x_{(i)}$	$dN(x_{(i)})$	$Y(x_{(i)})$	$\hat{S}(x_{(i)})$	I_1	I_2	$D_{i1,1}$	$D_{i1,2}$	$D_{i2,1}$	$D_{i2,2}$
1	0.326	1	10	0.90	1	1	0.100	0.010	0.100	0.010
2	1.158	1	9	0.80	1	1	0.111	0.022	0.111	0.022
3	1.715	1	8	0.70	1	1	0.125	0.038	0.125	0.038
4	2.832	1	7	0.60	0	1	0.143	0.058	0.000	0.038
5	3.087	0	6	0.60	0	1	0.000	0.058	0.000	0.038
6	3.231	1	5	0.48	0	1	0.200	0.098	0.000	0.038
7	3.289	1	4	0.36	0	1	0.250	0.161	0.000	0.038
8	3.294	1	3	0.24	0	1	0.333	0.272	0.000	0.038
9	3.371	1	2	0.12	0	0	0.000	0.272	0.000	0.038
10	3.985	0	1	0.12	0	0	0.000	0.272	0.000	0.038

Completing similar calculations for the other IDs, we have

$$\begin{aligned}\hat{e}(\hat{\theta}_{t_0}) &= (\hat{e}_1(\hat{\theta}_{t_0}),\ldots,\hat{e}_{10}(\hat{\theta}_{t_0})) \\ &= (.010,.010,.010,-.034,.001,-.038,-.035,-.028,.052,.052),\end{aligned}$$

which gives the variance estimate of $\hat{u}(\hat{\theta}_{t_0})$ as

$$\mathrm{Var}[\hat{u}(\hat{\theta}_{t_0})] \equiv \hat{\sigma}_{t_0}^2(\hat{\theta}_{t_0}) = \sum_{i=1}^{n} \hat{e}_i^2(\hat{\theta}_{t_0}) = 0.01.$$

Therefore 95% confidence interval for θ_{t_0} evaluated from (3.19) is $[1.24, \infty)$, which includes the true median residual lifetime at $t_0 = 2$, 1.42, evaluated from (3.20). This would be expected to happen for the 95% of the time. The open upper limit of this confidence interval is due to the small sample size. An increase of the sample size to 100 gives a tighter 95% confidence interval of $[0.81, 1.62]$.

To validate the procedure used in Table 3.3 to estimate (3.22), a simulation study was performed to assess type I error probabilities for testing the null hypothesis of 95% confidence intervals including the true median residual lifetime, which provided a close empirical type I error probability to the nominal level of 5%. This implies that it is important to include the cumulative information up to the censored observations in the test statistic as well, especially when the terms $D_{i1,2}$ and $D_{i2,2}$ are evaluated.

R codes used to generate the dataset and to perform data analysis presented in this example are provided in Appendix A.1.

3.5.2 Independent Two-Sample Case

Now suppose we are interested in comparing the median residual lifetimes between two groups at time t_0. Suppose that n_k ($k = 1, 2$) patients are randomized to a group k. Let $n = n_1 + n_2$. In group k, let T_{ki}, ($i = 1, \ldots, n_k$) be failure times with survivor function $S_k(t)$ and cumulative hazard function $H_k(t) = -\log S_k(t)$. In conjunction with failure time T_{ki}, let C_{ki} be the censoring time. Then, for a patient i from group k, we observe (X_{ki}, Δ_{ki}) ($i = 1, \ldots, n_k$), where $X_{ki} = \min(T_{ki}, C_{ki})$ and $\delta_{ki} = I(T_{ki} \leq C_{ki})$. Let $Y_{ki}(t) = I(X_{ki} \geq t)$ and $N_{ki}(t) = \Delta_{ki} I(X_{ki} \leq t)$ be the at-risk and death processes, respectively, for patient i in group k. We also define $Y_k(t) = \sum_{i=1}^{n_k} Y_{ki}(t)$ and $N_k(t) = \sum_{i=1}^{n_k} N_{ki}(t)$, and an associated martingale process $M_{ki}(t) = N_{ki}(t) - \int_0^t Y_{ki}(v) dH_k(v)$.

For group k, let $\hat{\theta}_{t_0}^{(k)}$ denote the sample estimate of the true median residual lifetime at time t_0, $\theta_{t_0,0}^{(k)}$. Note that $\hat{\theta}_{t_0}^{(k)}$ is nothing but the sample quantile of the conditional distribution of the residual lifetimes at time t_0, so that it is asymptotically a consistent estimator of the population quantile through the Bahadur representation given in (3.1) under the conditional distribution.

In general, comparison of two median residual lifetimes can be performed through either a difference or a ratio. Jeong *et al.* (2007) proposed to make inference based on the ratio of two median residual lifetimes, i.e. $r_{t_0} = \theta_{t_0,0}^{(2)}/\theta_{t_0,0}^{(1)}$. Investigators would often be interested in testing $H_0 : r_{t_0} = r_{t_0,0}$ vs. $H_1 : r_{t_0} \neq r_{t_0,0}$, where $r_{t_0,0}$ is a specified value of r_{t_0} under the null hypothesis. When $r_{t_0,0} = 1$ it will be tested whether two median residual lifetimes at a given time t_0 are equal or not. For group k, let the estimating function be

$$u_k(\theta_{t_0}^{(k)}) = \hat{S}_k(t_0 + \theta_{t_0}^{(k)}) - \frac{1}{2}\hat{S}_k(t_0).$$

In Sect. 3.5.1, we have shown that $u_k(\theta_{t_0}^{(k)})$ follows a normal distribution with mean 0 and variance $\sigma_{t_0}^2(\theta_{t_0}^{(k)})$, and hence the sample version of one-sample statistic $\hat{u}_k^2(\theta_{t_0}^{(k)})/\hat{\sigma}_{t_0}^2(\hat{\theta}_{t_0}^{(k)})$ follows a χ^2-distribution with 1 degree of freedom, which is extended to a two-sample case in the following theorem:

Theorem 4 (Jeong *et al.*, 2007). *Under the null hypothesis of $H_0 : r_{t_0} = r_{t_0,0}$, define a two-sample test statistic*

$$V_{t_0}(\theta_{t_0}^{(1)}, r_{t_0,0}) = \frac{u_1^2(\theta_{t_0}^{(1)})}{\hat{\sigma}_{t_0}^2(\hat{\theta}_{t_0}^{(1)})} + \frac{u_2^2(\theta_{t_0}^{(2)})}{\hat{\sigma}_{t_0}^2(\hat{\theta}_{t_0}^{(2)})} = \frac{u_1^2(\theta_{t_0}^{(1)})}{\hat{\sigma}_{t_0}^2(\hat{\theta}_{t_0}^{(1)})} + \frac{u_2^2(r_{t_0,0}\theta_{t_0}^{(1)})}{\hat{\sigma}_{t_0}^2(\hat{\theta}_{t_0}^{(2)})}.$$

Then statistic $W_{t_0}(r_{t_0,0}) = \min_{\theta_{t_0}^{(1)}} V_{t_0}(\theta_{t_0}^{(1)}, r_{t_0,0})$ follows asymptotically a χ_1^2-distribution with 1 degree of freedom.

Note that one way of eliminating the nuisance parameter $\theta_{t_0}^{(1)}$ in $V_{t_0}(\theta_{t_0}^{(1)}, r_{t_0,0})$ is to minimize it out, so that the statistic $W_{t_0}(r_{t_0,0})$ was referred to as the minimum dispersion statistic by Su and Wei (1993).

Proof. For group 1, at a value of $\theta_{t_0}^{(1)}$ in a small neighborhood around the true value $\theta_{t_0,0}^{(1)}$, we have

$$
\begin{aligned}
u_1\left(\theta_{t_0}^{(1)}\right) &= \hat{S}_1\left(t_0 + \theta_{t_0}^{(1)}\right) - \frac{1}{2}\hat{S}_1(t_0) \\
&= \hat{S}_1\left(t_0 + \theta_{t_0}^{(1)}\right) - S_1\left(t_0 + \theta_{t_0}^{(1)}\right) - \frac{1}{2}\left\{\hat{S}_1(t_0) - S_1(t_0)\right\},
\end{aligned}
$$

since $S_1\left(t_0 + \theta_{t_0}^{(1)}\right) - (1/2)S_1(t_0) = 0$ asymptotically.

Together with the asymptotic uniform consistency of the Kaplan–Meier estimator (Shorack and Wellner, 2009, Theorem

7.3.1, p. 304), Taylor series expansion of $u_1\left(\theta_{t_0}^{(1)}\right)$ at the estimate $\hat{\theta}_{t_0}^{(1)}$ gives

$$u_1\left(\theta_{t_0}^{(1)}\right) = -f_1\left(t_0 + \theta_{t_0,0}^{(1)}\right)\left(\hat{\theta}_{t_0}^{(1)} - \theta_{t_0}^{(1)}\right) + o_p\left(n^{-1/2}\right), \qquad (3.23)$$

where $f_k(\cdot)$ $(k = 1, 2)$ defines the probability density function of $S_k(\cdot)$.

Now let $r_{t_0} = \theta_{t_0,0}^{(2)}/\theta_{t_0,0}^{(1)}$ and $\hat{r}_{t_0} = \hat{\theta}_{t_0}^{(2)}/\hat{\theta}_{t_0}^{(1)}$. Then, similarly for group 2, we have

$$\begin{aligned}
u_2\left(\theta_{t_0}^{(1)}\right) &\equiv \hat{S}_2\left(t_0 + \theta_{t_0}^{(2)}\right) - \frac{1}{2}\hat{S}_2(t_0) \\
&= -f_2\left(t_0 + \theta_{t_0,0}^{(2)}\right)\left(\hat{\theta}_{t_0}^{(2)} - \theta_{t_0}^{(2)}\right) + o_p\left(n^{-1/2}\right) \\
&= -f_2\left(t_0 + \theta_{t_0,0}^{(2)}\right)\left\{\theta_{t_0,0}^{(1)}(\hat{r}_{t_0} - r_{t_0,0}) + r_{t_0,0}(\hat{\theta}_{t_0}^{(1)} - \theta_{t_0}^{(1)})\right\} \\
&\quad + o_p\left(n^{-1/2}\right),
\end{aligned} \qquad (3.24)$$

after applying the bivariate Taylor series expansion to $\hat{r}_{t_0}\hat{\theta}_{t_0}^{(1)}$ at $\left(r_{t_0,0}, \theta_{t_0,0}^{(1)}\right)$.

From (3.23) and (3.24), we have $V_{t_0}\left(r_{t_0,0}, \theta_{t_0}^{(1)}\right) = K_{t_0}\left(r_{t_0,0}, \theta_{t_0}^{(1)}\right)$ $+ o_p\left(n^{-1}\right)$, where

$$\begin{aligned}
K_{t_0}\left(r_{t_0,0}, \theta_{t_0}^{(1)}\right) &= \frac{u_1^2\left(\theta_{t_0}^{(1)}\right)}{\sigma_{t_0}^2\left(\theta_{t_0,0}^{(1)}\right)} + \frac{u_2^2\left(\theta_{t_0}^{(1)}\right)}{\sigma_{t_0}^2\left(\theta_{t_0,0}^{(2)}\right)} \\
&= \frac{f_1^2\left(t_0 + \theta_{t_0,0}^{(1)}\right)\left(\hat{\theta}_{t_0}^{(1)} - \theta_{t_0}^{(1)}\right)^2}{\sigma_1^2\left(\theta_{t_0,0}^{(1)}\right)} \\
&\quad + \frac{f_2^2\left(t_0 + \theta_{t_0,0}^{(2)}\right)\left\{\theta_{t_0,0}^{(1)}(\hat{r}_{t_0} - r_{t_0,0}) + r_{t_0,0}\left(\hat{\theta}_{t_0}^{(1)} - \theta_{t_0}^{(1)}\right)\right\}^2}{\sigma_2^2\left(\theta_{t_0,0}^{(2)}\right)}.
\end{aligned}$$

Therefore, minimizing $V_{t_0}\left(r_{t_0,0}, \theta_{t_0}^{(1)}\right)$ over $\theta_{t_0}^{(1)}$ is equivalent to minimizing the quadratic form $K_{t_0}\left(r_{t_0,0}, \theta_{t_0}^{(1)}\right)$, which occurs asymptotically at $\theta_{t_0}^{(1)} = \hat{\theta}_{t_0}^{(1)}$ because $\hat{\theta}_{t_0}^{(1)}$ is a consistent estimator of $\theta_{t_0,0}^{(1)}$ as well as $\theta_{t_0}^{(1)}$ converges to $\hat{\theta}_{t_0}^{(1)}$ as $n \to \infty$. This implies that for any arbitrary point $\theta_{t_0}^{(1)}$ close to the true value

$\theta_{t_0,0}^{(1)}$, $K_{t_0}\left(r_{t_0,0}, \theta_{t_0}^{(1)}\right)$ gets minimized at its estimate $\hat{\theta}_{t_0}^{(1)}$. Finally $K_{t_0}\left(r_{t_0,0}, \theta_{t_0}^{(1)}\right)$ asymptotically minimizes to

$$\frac{f_2^2\left(t_0 + \theta_{t_0,0}^{(2)}\right)\left\{\theta_{t_0,0}^{(1)}\right\}^2 (\hat{r}_{t_0} - r_{t_0,0})^2}{\sigma_2^2\left(\theta_{t_0,0}^{(2)}\right)},$$

which is equivalent to $(\hat{r} - r_0)^2/\mathrm{var}(\hat{r})$ from (3.24), following an asymptotic χ^2 distribution with 1 degree of freedom. This result still holds, by the Slutsky' theorem (Slutsky, 1925) , for the sample version of the two-sample test statistic $W_{t_0}(r_{t_0,0})$ by replacing the true parameters by their consistent estimators.

A large value of the statistic $W_{t_0}(r_{t_0,0})$ would reject the null hypothesis of $H_0 : r_{t_0} = r_{t_0,0}$, say if $W_{t_0}(r_{t_0,0}) > \chi_{1-\alpha,1}^2$ at the significance level of α. Also, a $100 \times (1 - \alpha)\%$ confidence interval for r_{t_0} can be constructed from

$$\{r_{t_0} : \inf_{\theta_{t_0}^{(1)}} V_{t_0}\left(r_{t_0}, \theta_{t_0}^{(1)}\right) < \chi_{1-\alpha,1}^2\}. \tag{3.25}$$

To obtain a confidence interval from (3.25), the statistic $V_{t_0}(r_{t_0}, \theta_{t_0}^{(1)})$ needs to be first minimized over $\theta_{t_0}^{(1)}$ for each fixed value of r_{t_0}. Then the minimum and maximum values of r_{t_0} associated with the values of the minimum statistic less than $\chi_{1-\alpha,1}^2$ will be the lower and upper limits of the confidence interval.

To accommodate heterogeneity in the population, a stratified test statistic can also be constructed. Denoting l to be the number of strata, the stratified test statistic can be formed as

$$A_{t_0}(r_{t_0,0}) = \sum_{j=1}^{l} W_{t_0}^{(j)}(r_{t_0,0}), \tag{3.26}$$

where $W_{t_0}^{(j)}(r_{t_0,0})$ is the statistic $W_{t_0}(r_{t_0,0})$ that corresponds to the jth stratum. The statistic $A_{t_0}(r_{t_0,0})$ will asymptotically follow a χ^2-distribution with l degrees of freedom.

Again the results developed for the two-sample median residual life inference can be easily extended to the τ-quantile residual lifetime simply by replacing the estimating equation for group k by

$$u_k(\theta_{t_0}^{(k)}) = \hat{S}_k(t_0 + \theta_{t_0}^{(k)}) - (1 - \tau)\hat{S}_k(t_0).$$

Example 3.4 (Numerical Calculation of Two-Sample Stati stic). In Example 3.3, we have demonstrated how to calculate one-sample test statistic numerically. For a two-sample case, we have generated two datasets for groups 1 and 2 from the same distribution used for one-sample case with a sample size of 100 for each group. Suppose we are interested in testing the null hypothesis of $H_0 : r_2 = 1$, where $r_2 = \theta_{2,0}^{(2)}/\theta_{2,0}^{(1)}$ is the ratio of two median residual lifetimes at a given time $t_0 = 2$. The estimated median residual lifetimes from the simulated dataset were $\hat{\theta}_2^{(1)} = 1.33$ for group 1 and $\hat{\theta}_2^{(2)} = 1.36$ for group 2, respectively, so that the estimated ratio was 1.02, close to 1 as expected. The variances of $\hat{u}_1(\hat{\theta}_2^{(1)})$ and $\hat{u}_2(\hat{\theta}_2^{(2)})$ can be calculated similarly as in Example 3.3. The test statistic $W_2(1)$ gives the value of $0.22 < \chi_{0.95,1}^2 = 3.841$, where $\chi_{0.95,1}^2$ is the 95th percentile of a χ^2-distribution with 1 degree of freedom, suggesting a lack of statistical evidence to reject the null hypothesis. Figure 3.6 shows the numerical evaluation of the statistic $W_2(r_2)$ as a function of r_2. A 95% confidence interval for r_2 can be obtained as (0.64, 1.62) by inverting the curve in Fig. 3.6 at the dashed line.

R codes used to generate the dataset and to perform data analysis presented in this example are provided in Appendix A.2.

Example 3.5 (Real Data Example). Jeong *et al.* (2007) considered a real data example from a phase III clinical trial on breast cancer treatment, referred to as NSABP B-04 data, where "NSABP" stands for National Surgical Adjuvant Breast and Bowel Project, a National Cancer Institute (NCI) cooperative group. In early to mid-1970s, the study was designed to compare two surgical procedures for breast cancer patients; radical mastectomy vs. total mastectomy, a less extensive surgery, with or without radiation therapy. A total of 1,079 women with negative axillary nodes were randomized to radical mastectomy, total mastectomy without axillary dissection but with post-operative irradiation, or

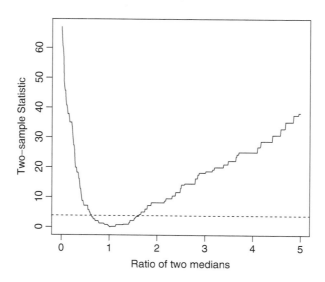

Fig. 3.6: Estimation of 95% confidence interval for r_2 by inverting two-sample test statistic when sample size is 100 per group

total mastectomy with axillary dissection if their nodes became positive. A total of 586 women with positive axillary nodes underwent either radical mastectomy or total mastectomy without axillary dissection but with post-operative irradiation. Fisher *et al.* (2002) reported an analysis of the 25-year follow-up update of the B-04 data. The long-term follow-up analysis confirmed that there was no significant difference between the two surgical procedures in terms of disease-free survival and overall survival. Therefore Jeong *et al.* (2007) used the nodal status as a significant group indicator in their analysis. The procedures discussed in Sects. 3.5.1 and 3.5.2 were applied to estimate the median residual lifetimes in node-positive and node-negative patients and 95% confidence interval for the ratio of the two median residual lifetimes at a given time point. Table 3.4 summarizes the results from Jeong *et al.* (2007).

In Table 3.4, for a node-negative woman, the median residual lifetime at 4 years after the surgery would be about 13 years whereas it would be 8 years for a node-positive woman. This can be used as the baseline information, if a new drug for secondary

Table 3.4: Estimated median residual lifetimes (MRL) in node-negative and node-positive groups, the ratios, and 95% confidence intervals for the ratios (NSABP B-04 data) [Jeong *et al.*, 2007, *Biometrics*]

	MRL		MRL ratio	95% CI
t_0	Node −	Node +		
0	12.46	6.87	0.55	(0.49, 0.63)
2	12.44	6.93	0.56	(0.47, 0.70)
4	13.05	8.24	0.63	(0.49, 0.81)
6	13.40	8.75	0.65	(0.54, 0.81)
8	12.91	10.19	0.79	(0.66, 0.93)
10	12.48	9.66	0.77	(0.62, 1.00)
12	11.85	9.66	0.82	(0.63, 1.08)

therapy is being tested during the follow-up period in terms of prolonging the remaining life years. The ratio of the two median residual life estimates at year 4 is 0.63 with 95% confidence interval (0.49,0.81), implying a significant difference between the two nodal groups in the median residual lifetime. Statistically significant difference in the median residual lifetimes sustains through about 10 years and then it fades away. This is a major advantage of the analysis based on the residual life, providing a panoramic view of the change in the population as time progresses.

3.6 Regression on Quantile Residual Life

In the previous section, we have considered a two-sample test statistic to compare the median, or quantile, residual lifetimes. In practice, however, the data analysis might benefit more from a regression modeling if a relationship between the quantile residual lifetimes and a continuous covariate such as age is investigated, or to adjust for possible confounding factors as covariates. In this section we consider a linear regression model for the τ-quantile of residual lifetimes at time t_0, on a log-scale,

$$\tau\text{-quantile}\{\log(T_i - t_0)|T_i > t_0, \mathbf{z}_i\} = \boldsymbol{\beta}'_{\tau|t_0}\mathbf{z}_i, \qquad (3.27)$$

where $\boldsymbol{\beta}_{\tau|t_0} = (\beta^{(0)}_{\tau|t_0}, \beta^{(1)}_{\tau|t_0}, \ldots, \beta^{(p)}_{\tau|t_0})'$ denotes a vector of the regression coefficients, and $\mathbf{z}_i = (1, z_{1i}, \ldots, z_{pi})'$ is a vector of covariates for a subject i. The model (3.27) specifies a linear relationship between the τ-quantile residual lifetimes on a log-scale and the vector of covariates at a *specific* time t_0, allowing for testing, say, a group effect adjusting for other covariates.

To examine interpretation of the regression parameters under the model (3.27), let us consider a simple median residual life regression model

$$\text{median}\{\log(T_i - t_0)|T_i > t_0, z_{1i}\} = \beta^{(0)}_{t_0} + \beta^{(1)}_{t_0}z_{1i}, \qquad (3.28)$$

where z_{1i} is a binary covariate, say, 0 for the control group and 1 for an intervention group. Here $\beta^{(k)}_{t_0}$ $(k = 0, 1)$ denotes the regression coefficients for the intercept $(k = 0)$ and slope $(k = 1)$ at time t_0. By the invariance property of the median with respect to monotone transformations, the model (3.28) is equivalent to

$$\text{median}(T_i - t_0|T_i > t_0, z_{1i}) = \exp(\beta^{(0)}_{t_0} + \beta^{(1)}_{t_0}z_{1i}).$$

Therefore $\exp(\beta^{(0)}_{t_0})$ and $\exp(\beta^{(0)}_{t_0} + \beta^{(1)}_{t_0})$ can be interpreted as the median residual lifetimes for the control and intervention groups at time t_0, respectively, so that the difference in median residual lifetime between the two groups is given by

$$\exp(\beta^{(0)}_{t_0})\{\exp(\beta^{(1)}_{t_0}) - 1\}.$$

In this case, the slope parameter $\beta^{(1)}_{t_0}$ can be interpreted as the logarithm of the *ratio* of the two median residual lifetimes at time point t_0.

3.6.1   Parametric Estimation of Regression Parameters

For the *conditional* parametric inference on the effects of the covariates on the quantile residual life, let us consider a simple log-linear model

$$\tau\text{-quantile}\{\log(T_i^*)|T_i > t_0, z_i\} = \beta^{(0)}_{\tau|t_0} + \beta^{(1)}_{\tau|t_0}z_i + \sigma W_i, \qquad (3.29)$$

where $T_i^* = T_i - t_0$ and W_i's follow an error distribution that can take a parametric form such as Weibull, log-logistic, or Pareto. Denoting $S_{t_0}^*(t|z)$ for the survival function of the residual lifetime T_i^* given $T_i > t_0$ and the covariate z, the log-linear model (3.29) is equivalent to the accelerated failure time (AFT) model

$$S_{t_0}^*(t|z_i) = S_{t_0,0}^*\left(t\exp(-\beta_{\tau|t_0}^{(1)} z_i)\right),$$

since

$$
\begin{aligned}
S_{t_0}^*(t|z_i) &= \Pr(T_i^* > t|z_i) \\
&= \Pr\left(\exp(\beta_{\tau|t_0}^{(0)} + \beta_{\tau|t_0}^{(1)} z_i + \sigma W_i) > t\right) \\
&= \Pr\left(\exp(\beta_{\tau|t_0}^{(0)} + \sigma W_i) > t\exp(-\beta_{\tau|t_0}^{(1)} z_i)\right) \\
&= S_{t_0,0}^*\left(t\exp(-\beta_{\tau|t_0}^{(1)} z_i)\right),
\end{aligned}
\tag{3.30}
$$

where $S_{t_0,0}^*(\cdot)$ is the baseline survival function for $T_i^* = \exp\left(\beta_{\tau|t_0}^{(0)} + \sigma W_i\right)$. Here note that the signs of the regression coefficients have been reversed. Furthermore, when the distribution of W_i's is given by the standard extreme value distribution with the survival function $S_W(w) = \exp(-\exp(w))$, we have

$$
\begin{aligned}
S_{t_0}^*(t|z_i) &= S_{t_0,0}^*\left(t\exp(-\beta_{\tau|t_0}^{(1)} z_i)\right) \\
&= \exp\left[-\exp\left\{\frac{\log\left(t\exp(-\beta_{\tau|t_0}^{(1)} z_i)\right) - \beta_{\tau|t_0}^{(0)}}{\sigma}\right\}\right] \\
&= \left[\exp\left\{-\exp\left(\frac{\log(t) - \beta_{\tau|t_0}^{(0)}}{\sigma}\right)\right\}\right]^{\exp\left(-\beta_{\tau|t_0}^{(1)} z_i/\sigma\right)} \\
&= S_{t_0,0}^*(t)^{\exp\left(-\beta_{\tau|t_0}^{(1)} z_i/\sigma\right)},
\end{aligned}
$$

because, without covariates, we have

$$
\begin{aligned}
S_{t_0,0}^*(t) &= \Pr(T_i^* > t) = \Pr\left(\exp(\beta_{\tau|t_0}^{(0)} + \sigma W_i) > t\right) \\
&= \Pr\left(W_i > \left(\log(t) - \beta_{\tau|t_0}^{(0)}\right)/\sigma\right) \\
&= S_W\left(\left(\log(t) - \beta_{\tau|t_0}^{(0)}\right)/\sigma\right) \\
&= \exp\left[-\exp\left(\frac{\log(t) - \beta_{\tau|t_0}^{(0)}}{\sigma}\right)\right] \\
&= \exp\left[-\exp\left\{-\left(\beta_{\tau|t_0}^{(0)}\right)/\sigma\right\} t^{1/\sigma}\right].
\end{aligned}
$$

This implies that the log-linear quantile residual life regression model, or equivalently, the AFT model for the residual life distribution, reduces to the proportional hazards model with the proportionality parameter $\exp\left(-\beta_{\tau|t_0}^{(1)} z_i/\sigma\right)$. In this case, the baseline distribution of T_i^* follows a Weibull distribution with the survival function of $S(t) = \exp(-\lambda t^\kappa)$ where $\kappa = 1/\sigma$ is a shape parameter and $\lambda = e^{-\beta_{\tau|t_0}^{(0)}/\sigma}$ is a rate parameter. Similarly, when the distribution of W's follows the standard logistic distribution with the survival function $S_W(w) = 1/(1+\exp(w))$, it reduces to the proportional odds model with the proportionality parameter $\exp\left(\beta_{\tau|t_0}^{(1)} z_i/\sigma\right)$. The baseline distribution of the residual lifetime T_i^* for this case would be the log-logistic distribution with the survival function $S(t) = 1/(1 + \lambda t^\kappa)$ where κ and λ were defined above.

Now the general formula for the τ-quantile residual lifetime can be derived regardless of any parametric assumption for the error distribution. As also noted earlier, the conditional survival function of the random variable T_i^* given a covariate z_i at time t_0 is

$$
\begin{aligned}
S_{t_0}^*(t|z_i) &= \Pr(T_i^* > t|z) = \Pr\left(\exp\left(\beta_{\tau|t_0}^{(0)} + \beta_{\tau|t_0}^{(1)} z_i + \sigma W_i\right) > t\right) \\
&= \Pr\left(W_i > \frac{\log(t) - \beta_{\tau|t_0}^{(0)} - \beta_{\tau|t_0}^{(1)} z_i}{\sigma}\right) \\
&= S_W\left(\frac{\log(t) - \beta_{\tau|t_0}^{(0)} - \beta_{\tau|t_0}^{(1)} z_i}{\sigma}\right).
\end{aligned}
$$

Note that the τ-quantile residual life function given the co-variate z_i under the distribution of T_i^*, $\theta_{\tau|t_0}(z_i)$, is given by

$$\theta_{\tau|t_0}(z_i) = S_{t_0}^{*-1}(1-\tau) = \exp\left(\sigma S_W^{-1}(1-\tau) + \beta_{\tau|t_0}^{(0)} + \beta_{\tau|t_0}^{(1)} z_i\right),$$
$$(3.31)$$

because

$$\Pr(T_i - t_0 > \theta_{\tau|t_0}(z_i)|T_i > t_0; z_i) = 1 - \tau$$

implies

$$\frac{S_{t_0}^{*-1}(\theta_{\tau|t_0}(z_i))}{S_{t_0}^{*-1}(0)} = 1 - \tau$$

and

$$S_{t_0}^{*-1}(x|z_i) = \exp\left(\sigma S_W^{-1}(x) + \beta_{\tau|t_0}^{(0)} + \beta_{\tau|t_0}^{(1)} z_i\right).$$

Equation (3.31) can be further specified once the distribution of W's is determined as shown in the following example.

Example 3.6. Suppose that the error distribution of the residual lifetimes T_i^* at time t_0 follows the standard extreme value distribution with the survival function $S_W(w) = \exp(-\exp(w))$, which has the inverse function as $S_W^{-1}(x) = \log\{-\log(x)\}$. Therefore the τ-quantile residual lifetime at time t_0 in (3.31) simplifies to

$$\theta_{\tau|t_0}(z_i) = \exp\left(\beta_{\tau|t_0}^{(0)} + \beta_{\tau|t_0}^{(1)} z_i\right)\{-\log(1-\tau)\}^\sigma.$$

Note that when there is no covariate, this reduces to $\lambda^{-1/\kappa}\{-\log(1-\tau)\}^{1/\kappa}$, which is the τ-quantile residual life function for the Weibull distribution with $\kappa = 1/\sigma$ and $\lambda = e^{-\beta_{\tau|t_0}^{(0)}/\sigma}$ without t_0.

Similarly when we have the error distribution of the standard logistic distribution with the survival function $S_W(w) = 1/(1+e^w)$ with its inverse function $S_W^{-1}(x) = \log(1/x - 1)$, the τ-quantile residual lifetime at time t_0 is given by

$$\theta_{\tau|t_0}(z_i) = \exp\left(\beta_{\tau|t_0}^{(0)} + \beta_{\tau|t_0}^{(1)} z_i\right)\left\{\frac{\tau}{1-\tau}\right\}^\sigma.$$

Again, without the covariate, this reduces to $\lambda^{-1/\kappa}\{\tau/(1-\tau)\}^{1/\kappa}$, which is the τ-quantile residual life function for the log-logistic distribution with $\kappa = 1/\sigma$ and $\lambda = e^{-\beta_{\tau|t_0}^{(0)}/\sigma}$ without t_0.

To estimate $\theta_{\tau|t_0}(z_i)$, the parameters σ, $\beta_{\tau|t_0}^{(0)}$, and $\beta_{\tau|t_0}^{(1)}$ can be replaced by their maximum likelihood estimators by the in-variance property. Let us denote C_i for the potential censoring time, so that $X_i^* = \min(T_i^*, C_i)$ is the observed residual lifetime T_i^* at t_0, and $\delta_i^* = I(T_i^* \le C_i)$. For parametric inference for the observed right-censored data $\{(X_i^*, \delta_i^*, z_i), i = 1, \ldots, n\}$, the likelihood function is given by

$$L(\beta_{\tau|t_0}^{(0)}, \beta_{\tau|t_0}^{(1)}, \sigma) = \prod_{i=1}^{n} [f_{t_0}^*(x_i^*|z_i)]^{\delta_i^*} [S_{t_0}^*(x_i^*|z_i)]^{1-\delta_i^*}$$

$$= \prod_{i=1}^{n} \left[\frac{1}{\sigma x_i^*} f_W \left(\frac{\log(x_i^*) - \beta_{\tau|t_0}^{(0)} - \beta_{\tau|t_0}^{(1)} z_i}{\sigma} \right) \right]^{\delta_i^*}$$

$$\times \left[S_W \left(\frac{\log(x_i^*) - \beta_{\tau|t_0}^{(0)} - \beta_{\tau|t_0}^{(1)} z_i}{\sigma} \right) \right]^{1-\delta_i^*}, \qquad (3.32)$$

where $f_W(v|z_i) = -(d/dv)S_W(v|z_i)$. The maximum likelihood estimators for σ, $\beta_{\tau|t_0}^{(0)}$, and $\beta_{\tau|t_0}^{(1)}$ can be obtained by maximizing the likelihood function (3.32) via an optimization algorithm such as the Newton–Raphson. The variances of those estimators can be achieved from the inverse of the observed information matrix whose elements will be the negative second derivatives with respect to the parameters, evaluated at the observed data and the parameter estimates. As mentioned earlier, the τ-quantile resid-ual lifetime at time t_0 given some covariate values, $\theta_{\tau|t_0}(z_i)$, can be estimated by replacing the parameters in (3.31) with their estimates. The variance of the estimated τ-quantile residual life $\hat{\theta}_{\tau|t_0}(z_i)$ can be evaluated by applying the tri-variate delta method.

3.6.2   "Setting the Clock Back to 0" Property

In the previous section, we have considered parametric inference on the log-linear model of the quantile residual life by assuming a specific parametric form for the residual life distribution condi-tional on a given time point t_0. We have shown that the log-linear regression model is equivalent to the AFT regression model with the signs of the regression parameters reversed, which gives the proportional hazards model with Weibull baseline and proportional odds model with log-logistic baseline as special cases with the standard extreme value error distribution and the standard logistic error distribution, respectively. One legitimate concern for the parametric inference on the regression model for the residual lifetimes could be that the family of the residual life distribution might change over time, so that the parametric assumption for the baseline residual life distribution might be violated, resulting in invalid analysis results. It would be useful if a family of distributions can be identified, which has the distribution invariance property over time, referred to as "setting the clock back to zero" (SCBZ) property studied by Rao *et al.* (1993). In this section, we review the main results from Rao *et al.* (1993).

Definiton 3.2 (Setting the Clock Back to Zero Property).
Suppose $S(t, \psi)$ is the survival function of the random variable T determined by the parameter vector ψ and $S(t + t_0, \psi)$ is the survival function of the residual life distribution at time t_0. The family of survival functions $S(t, \psi)$ ($\psi \in \Omega$, where Ω is a parameter space) is said to have "SCBZ" property or said to be invariant if the following equation holds:

$$\Pr(T > t + t_0 | T > t_0, \psi) = \Pr(T > t, \psi^*),$$

or

$$\frac{S(t + t_0, \psi)}{S(t_0, \psi)} = S(t, \psi^*), \tag{3.33}$$

where $S(t, \psi^*)$ is the survival function of the same distribution as T, with an updated parameter vector ψ^*. This implies that the residual life distribution remains in the same family as the initial distribution.

Two well-known distributions, Pareto and Gompertz, have the SCBZ property as illustrated in the following examples.

Example 3.7 (Pareto). Suppose the initial distribution of T follows the Pareto distribution with the survival function of $S(t, \psi) = (1 + \lambda t)^{-\kappa}$ ($\lambda > 0, \kappa > 1$), so that $\psi = (\lambda, \kappa)$ is a vector of the parameters. Under this distribution, the left-hand side of Eq. (3.33), the residual life survival function, gives

$$\frac{S(t + t_0, \boldsymbol{\psi})}{S(t_0, \boldsymbol{\psi})} = \left\{ \frac{1 + \lambda(t + t_0)}{1 + \lambda t_0} \right\}^{-\kappa} = S(t, \boldsymbol{\psi}^*),$$

where $\boldsymbol{\psi}^* = (\lambda(1 + \lambda t_0)^{-1}, \kappa)$, so that the Pareto distribution family enjoys the SCBZ property.

Example 3.8 (Gompertz). Let us consider the family of the Gompertz distribution (Gompertz, 1825) with the survival function of

$$S(t, \boldsymbol{\psi}) = \exp \left\{ -(\kappa/\lambda) \left(e^{\lambda t} - 1 \right) \right\},$$

where $\boldsymbol{\psi} = (\lambda, \kappa)$ $(-\infty < \lambda < \infty, 0 < \kappa < \infty)$. With this survival function, the conditional residual life survival function is given by

$$
\begin{aligned}
\frac{S(t + t_0, \boldsymbol{\psi})}{S(t_0, \boldsymbol{\psi})} &= \exp \left[-(\kappa/\lambda) \left\{ e^{\lambda(t + t_0)} - e^{\lambda t_0} \right\} \right] \\
&= \exp \left[-(\kappa e^{\lambda t_0}/\lambda) \left\{ e^{\lambda t} - 1 \right\} \right] = S(t, \boldsymbol{\psi}^*),
\end{aligned}
$$

where $\boldsymbol{\psi}^* = (\lambda, \kappa e^{\lambda t_0})$. An important feature of the Gompertz is that it can model an improper distribution that can be useful for the cure fraction or competing risks analysis.

Another distribution that has the SCBZ property is the extended exponential family with the survival function $S(t, \boldsymbol{\psi}) = \exp \left[- \{ \lambda t + (\kappa/2) t^2 \} \right]$, where $\boldsymbol{\psi} = (\lambda, \kappa)$ $(\lambda > 0, \kappa \geq 0)$. Note that this reduces to an exponential distribution with the rate parameter λ when $\kappa = 0$. Unfortunately, though, some popular parametric distributions in survival analysis such as Weibull and log-logistic do not enjoy this property.

This result is extended to the AFT regression model in the following theorem:

Theorem 5 (Rao *et al.*, 1993). *The family of the survival distributions under the AFT model has the SCBZ property if the family of the baseline survival distributions of the AFT regression model has the SCBZ property.*

Proof: *Necessity.* Suppose we have the AFT regression model $S(t, \boldsymbol{\psi}|z) = S_0(\eta t, \boldsymbol{\psi})$, where $\eta = \exp(-\beta z)$ for the notational consistency with (3.30). Note that β could be a vector of the regression parameters from the original log-linear residual life regression model (3.29). By the assumption, we have

$$\frac{S(t + t_0, \boldsymbol{\psi}|z)}{S(t_0, \boldsymbol{\psi}|z)} = S(t, \boldsymbol{\psi}^*|z),$$

which, under the AFT model, implies that

$$\frac{S_0(t^* + t_0^*, \boldsymbol{\psi})}{S_0(t_0^*, \boldsymbol{\psi})} = S_0(t^*, \boldsymbol{\psi}^*),$$

where $t^* = \eta t$ and $t_0^* = \eta t_0$, implying the SCBZ property holds for the baseline residual life distribution.

Sufficiency. If the SCBZ property holds for the baseline conditional residual life distribution under the AFT regression model, we have

$$\frac{S(t + t_0, \boldsymbol{\psi}|z)}{S(t_0, \boldsymbol{\psi}|z)}) = \frac{S_0(t^* + t_0^*, \boldsymbol{\psi})}{S_0(t_0^*, \boldsymbol{\psi})} = S_0(t^*, \boldsymbol{\psi}^*) = S(t, \boldsymbol{\psi}^*|z),$$

which implies that if the baseline residual life distribution is closed under the SCBZ property, so does the residual life distribution adjusted for the covariates under the AFT model.

When a family of the baseline distributions under the log-linear quantile residual life regression model (3.29), or equivalently under the corresponding AFT regression model, has the SCBZ property, then it is straightforward to estimate the quantile residual lifetime at any time point given some covariate values through the parameter estimates from the initial distribution. To see this, the τ-quantile residual lifetime at t_0, $\theta_{\tau|t_0}$, under the AFT regression model can be estimated from

$$\Pr(T > t_0 + \theta_{\tau|t_0}|T > t_0, z, \boldsymbol{\psi}) = 1 - \tau,$$

or equivalently

$$\frac{S(T > t_0 + \theta_{\tau|t_0}, \boldsymbol{\psi}|z)}{S(T > t_0, \boldsymbol{\psi}|z)} = 1 - \tau.$$

Now by the AFT assumption and the SCBZ property of the baseline distributions, we have

$$\frac{S_0(T > \eta(t_0 + \theta_{\tau|t_0}), \boldsymbol{\psi}|z)}{S_0(T > \eta t_0, \boldsymbol{\psi}|z)} = 1 - \tau = S_0(\eta\theta_{\tau|t_0}, \boldsymbol{\psi}^*),$$

so that the τ-quantile residual life adjusted for covariates under the AFT regression model can be expressed as

$$\theta_{\tau|t_0}(z) = (1/\eta)S_0^{-1}(1 - \tau, \boldsymbol{\psi}^*), \tag{3.34}$$

where $\eta = \exp(-\beta z)$.

Example 3.9 (Pareto). When we have the Pareto distribution as the baseline with $S_0(t, \boldsymbol{\psi}) = (1 + \lambda t)^{-\kappa}$, recall that the resulting survival function for the residual lifetime at t_0 belongs to the Pareto distribution, with an updated rate parameter $\lambda^* = \lambda(1 + \lambda t_0)^{-1}$. Since $S_0^{-1}(x, \lambda^*, \kappa) = (1/\lambda^*)(x^{-1/\kappa} - 1)$, Eq. (3.34) gives

$$\theta_{\tau|t_0}(z) = (1/\eta)S_0^{-1}(1 - \tau, \lambda^*, \kappa) = \frac{1 + \lambda t_0}{\eta\lambda}\left\{(1 - \tau)^{-1/\kappa} - 1\right\}.$$

Example 3.10 (Gompertz). Similarly when the baseline distribution follows the Gompertz distribution with $S_0(t, \boldsymbol{\psi}) = \exp\left\{-(\kappa/\lambda)\left(e^{\lambda t} - 1\right)\right\}$, the resulting survival function for the residual lifetime at t_0 again belongs to the Gompertz distribution, with an updated shape parameter $\kappa^* = \kappa e^{\lambda t_0}$. Since $S_0^{-1}(x, \lambda, \kappa^*) = (1/\lambda)\log\{1 - (\lambda/\kappa^*)\log(x)\}$, we have the τ-quantile residual life at t_0 given covariates as

$$\begin{aligned}\theta_{\tau|t_0}(z) &= (1/\eta)S_0^{-1}(1 - \tau, \lambda, \kappa^*)\\ &= (1/\eta\lambda)\log\{1 - (\lambda e^{-\lambda t_0}/\kappa)\log(1 - \tau)\}.\end{aligned}$$

From the previous examples, one can see that once the SCBZ property of the baseline distributions under the log-linear quantile residual life regression model holds, the τ-quantile residual lifetime can be estimated based on the parameter estimates from the likelihood function formed for the initial distribution, together with the variance estimation by using the delta method.

When the SCBZ assumption is satisfied, it would be more efficient to use the Pareto or Gompertz distribution for the baseline for the parametric inference on the quantile residual lifetime through the AFT regression model than using the Weibull or log-logistic distribution.

3.6.3 Semiparametric Regression

In the previous section, we have considered a parametric inference procedure for the regression parameters from the log-linear regression model on the τ-quantile residual lifetimes given in (3.27). Here we review a semiparametric procedure (Jung *et al.*, 2009) for the regression parameters assuming an arbitrary error distribution.

First we derive an estimating equation for the median residual lifetime based on the least absolute deviation (LAD) between the residual life on a log-scale and the linear predictor. Suppose T_i denotes failure time without censoring. Then finding the median of the residual lifetimes on a log-scale as the linear function of the covariates requires minimization of $A(\boldsymbol{\beta}_{t_0})$ over $\boldsymbol{\beta}_{t_0}$, where

$$
\begin{aligned}
A(\boldsymbol{\beta}_{t_0}) &\equiv \sum_{i=1}^{n} |\log(T_i - t_0) - \boldsymbol{\beta}_{t_0}' \mathbf{z}_i| \\
&= \sum_{i=1}^{n} \Big[\{\log(T_i - t_0) - \boldsymbol{\beta}_{t_0}' \mathbf{z}_i\} I\{\log(T_i - t_0) - \boldsymbol{\beta}_{t_0}' \mathbf{z}_i > 0\} \\
&\qquad - \{\log(T_i - t_0) - \boldsymbol{\beta}_{t_0}' \mathbf{z}_i\} I\{\log(T_i - t_0) - \boldsymbol{\beta}_{t_0}' \mathbf{z}_i < 0\} \Big] \\
&= \sum_{i=1}^{n} \Big[\{\log(T_i - t_0) - \boldsymbol{\beta}_{t_0}' \mathbf{z}_i\} I\{\log(T_i - t_0) - \boldsymbol{\beta}_{t_0}' \mathbf{z}_i > 0\} \\
&\qquad - \{\log(T_i - t_0) - \boldsymbol{\beta}_{t_0}' \mathbf{z}_i\} [1 - I\{\log(T_i - t_0) - \boldsymbol{\beta}_{t_0}' \mathbf{z}_i > 0\}] \Big] \\
&= \sum_{i=1}^{n} \Big[2\{\log(T_i - t_0) - \boldsymbol{\beta}_{t_0}' \mathbf{z}_i\} I\{\log(T_i - t_0) - \boldsymbol{\beta}_{t_0}' \mathbf{z}_i > 0\} \\
&\qquad - \{\log(T_i - t_0) - \boldsymbol{\beta}_{t_0}' \mathbf{z}_i\} \Big] \\
&= 2 \sum_{i=1}^{n} \{\log(T_i - t_0) - \boldsymbol{\beta}_{t_0}' \mathbf{z}_i\} [I\{\log(T_i - t_0) - \boldsymbol{\beta}_{t_0}' \mathbf{z}_i > 0\} - 1/2],
\end{aligned}
$$

where the indicator function $I(T_i > t_0)$ was omitted for notational convenience. Note that the absolute function was defined as $f(x) = |x| = -x$ if $x < 0$ and x if $x > 0$, so that $1 - I(x < 0) = I(x > 0)$.

For the τ-quantile, this can be generalized to

$$\left(\frac{1}{1-\tau}\right) \sum_{i=1}^{n} \{\log(T_i - t_0) - \boldsymbol{\beta}'_{\tau|t_0}\mathbf{z}_i\}[I\{\log(T_i - t_0) - \boldsymbol{\beta}'_{\tau|t_0}\mathbf{z}_i > 0\} - (1 - \tau)]$$

$$= \left(\frac{1}{1-\tau}\right) \sum_{i=1}^{n} \{\log(T_i - t_0) - \boldsymbol{\beta}'_{\tau|t_0}\mathbf{z}_i\}[\tau - I\{\log(T_i - t_0) - \boldsymbol{\beta}'_{\tau|t_0}\mathbf{z}_i < 0\}]$$

$$= \left(\frac{1}{1-\tau}\right) \sum_{i=1}^{n} \rho_\tau(u_i), \qquad (3.35)$$

where $u_i = \log(T_i - t_0) - \boldsymbol{\beta}'_{\tau|t_0}\mathbf{z}_i$ and $\rho_\tau(u_i) = u_i(\tau - I(u_i < 0))$ is the check function defined in (1.9). By taking the first derivative of $A(\boldsymbol{\beta}_{\tau|t_0})$ with respect to $\boldsymbol{\beta}_{\tau|t_0}$, the estimating equation is given by $U(\boldsymbol{\beta}_{\tau|t_0}) = 0$, where

$$U(\boldsymbol{\beta}_{\tau|t_0}) = -\left(\frac{1}{1-\tau}\right) \sum_{i=1}^{n} \mathbf{z}_i[I\{\log(T_i - t_0) - \boldsymbol{\beta}'_{\tau|t_0}\mathbf{z}_i > 0\} - (1 - \tau)]$$

$$= -\left(\frac{1}{1-\tau}\right) \sum_{i=1}^{n} \mathbf{z}_i[I\{T_i > t_0 + \exp(\boldsymbol{\beta}'_{\tau|t_0}\mathbf{z}_i)\} - (1 - \tau)]$$

$$= \left(\frac{1}{1-\tau}\right) \sum_{i=1}^{n} \mathbf{z}_i[\tau - I\{T_i < t_0 + \exp(\boldsymbol{\beta}'_{\tau|t_0}\mathbf{z}_i)\}]$$

$$= \left(\frac{1}{1-\tau}\right) \sum_{i=1}^{n} \mathbf{z}_i\psi_\tau(u_i), \qquad (3.36)$$

where $\psi_\tau(u_i) = \tau - I(u_i < 0)$ is the first derivative of the check function.

Now suppose C_i is the potential censoring time, and let $X_i = \min(T_i, C_i)$ be the observed survival time. Assuming conditional independence between T_i and C_i given $\mathbf{z}_i$ and independence of C_i from $\mathbf{z}_i$, the following is true for the censored data,

$$E[I\{\log(X_i - t_0) > \boldsymbol{\beta}^{0'}_{\tau|t_0}\mathbf{z}_i\}|\mathbf{z}_i] = P\{X_i > t_0 + \exp(\boldsymbol{\beta}^{0'}_{\tau|t_0}\mathbf{z}_i)|\mathbf{z}_i\}$$

$$= P\{T_i > t_0 + \exp(\boldsymbol{\beta}^{0'}_{\tau|t_0}\mathbf{z}_i)|\mathbf{z}_i\}$$

$$\times P\{C_i > t_0 + \exp(\boldsymbol{\beta}^{0'}_{\tau|t_0}\mathbf{z}_i)|\mathbf{z}_i\},$$

which is equivalent to

$$\frac{P\{T_i > t_0 + \exp(\boldsymbol{\beta}_{\tau|t_0}^{0\prime}\mathbf{z}_i)|\mathbf{z}_i\}}{P(T_i > t_0|\mathbf{z}_i)}P(T_i > t_0|\mathbf{z}_i)P\{C_i > t_0 + \exp(\boldsymbol{\beta}_{\tau|t_0}^{0\prime}\mathbf{z}_i)\}.$$

Under the model (3.27) and by definition of the τ-quantile residual life function

$$\frac{P\{T_i > t_0 + \exp(\boldsymbol{\beta}_{\tau|t_0}^{0\prime}\mathbf{z}_i)|\mathbf{z}_i\}}{P(T_i > t_0|\mathbf{z}_i)} = 1 - \tau.$$

Therefore,

$$E[I\{\log(X_i - t_0) > \boldsymbol{\beta}_{\tau|t_0}^{0\prime}\mathbf{z}_i\}|\mathbf{z}_i]$$

$$= (1 - \tau)\frac{G\{t_0 + \exp(\boldsymbol{\beta}_{\tau|t_0}^{0\prime}\mathbf{z}_i)\}}{G(t_0)}P(X_i > t_0|\mathbf{z}_i)$$

$$= E\left[(1 - \tau)\frac{G\{t_0 + \exp(\boldsymbol{\beta}_{\tau|t_0}^{0\prime}\mathbf{z}_i)\}}{G(t_0)}I(X_i > t_0)\middle|\mathbf{z}_i\right],$$

and the following can be used as an estimating equation for the regression parameter $\boldsymbol{\beta}_{\tau|t_0}$,

$$\mathbf{S}_{\tau|t_0,n}(\boldsymbol{\beta}_{\tau|t_0}) = \sum_{i=1}^{n}\mathbf{z}_i\left[\frac{I\{X_i > t_0 + \exp(\boldsymbol{\beta}_{\tau|t_0}'\mathbf{z}_i)\}}{\hat{G}\{t_0 + \exp(\boldsymbol{\beta}_{\tau|t_0}'\mathbf{z}_i)\}}\right.$$
$$\left. -(1 - \tau)\frac{I(X_i > t_0)}{\hat{G}(t_0)}\right] \approx 0. \qquad (3.37)$$

Equation (3.37) reduces to one derived for the noncensored case given in (3.36), omitting the term $-1/(1 - \tau)$ and recalling that the indicator function $I(T_i > t_0)$ was suppressed in the latter.

Jung *et al.* (2009, Web Appendix A) showed that under certain regularity conditions, a solution $\hat{\boldsymbol{\beta}}_{\tau|t_0}$ to the estimating equation (3.37) is a consistent estimator of its true value $\boldsymbol{\beta}_{\tau|t_0}^{0}$. Once the regression parameters $\boldsymbol{\beta}_{\tau|t_0}$ are estimated from this equation, the median residual lifetime conditional on some covariate values can be estimated by $\exp(\hat{\boldsymbol{\beta}}_{\tau|t_0}'\mathbf{z}_i)$, where $\hat{\boldsymbol{\beta}}_{\tau|t_0}'$ is the LAD estimate of $\boldsymbol{\beta}_{\tau|t_0}'$.

Note that by the invariance property of the quantile with respect to monotone transformations, the estimating equation (3.37) can be evaluated on the original scale of the observed survival data, although the model (3.27) is based on a log-scale. The estimator $\hat{\beta}_{\tau|t_0}$ may be a minimizer of the function $\left\|\mathbf{S}_{\tau|t_0,n}(\beta_{\tau|t_0})\right\|$, where $\|\cdot\|$ is often defined as the square root of sum of squares. For the non-censored case, the regression parameters can be easily estimated from Eq. (3.36) by using the unit weights in `rq.wfit` which was used in the procedure `WRegEst` from the R package `emplik`. Under censoring, however, a dynamic grid search method can be used like throwing a fish net. First, a net of coarse grids is set up over the parameter space around some reasonable initial guesses and find the parameter values along the grid points that minimize the estimating equation close to 0. Next, a finer net of grids is set up around the parameter values achieved from the previous step and again obtain the updated parameter values that minimize the estimating equation close to 0, and so on. The size of the grid net can be reduced as the steps progress to shorten the computing time. However, as the number of covariates increases, the grid search method could be overly time-consuming, so that a more efficient optimization procedure needs to be developed for the estimating equation (3.37).

An alternative estimating equation can be formulated by further noticing in (3.36) that

$$E[\mathbf{z}g_\beta(T)|\mathbf{z}] = \int_0^\infty \mathbf{z}g_\beta(T)dF(T|\mathbf{z}) = 0, \qquad (3.38)$$

where

$$g_\beta(T) = I(T > t_0)[\tau - I\{T \le t_0 + \exp(\beta'_{\tau|t_0}\mathbf{z})\}],$$

because

$$
\begin{aligned}
E[\mathbf{z}g_\beta(T)|\mathbf{z}] &= \mathbf{z}E\left[I(T > t_0)[\tau - I\{T \le t_0 + \exp(\beta'_{\tau|t_0}\mathbf{z})\}]|\mathbf{z}\right] \\
&= -\mathbf{z}\left[(1-\tau)S(t_0) - S(t_0 + \exp(\beta'_{\tau|t_0}\mathbf{z}))\right] = 0,
\end{aligned}
$$

by the definition of the τ-quantile residual lifetime at t_0 under the model (3.27).

Based on the observed data, the expectation in (3.38) can be rewritten as

$$\sum_{i=1}^{n} \mathbf{z}_i g_\beta(X_i) d\hat{F}(X_i|\mathbf{z}_i),$$

where $d\hat{F}(X_i|\mathbf{z}) \equiv \Delta_i$ is the estimated probability mass function for the non-censored case at X_i and a jump of the Kaplan–Meier estimates based on (X_i, δ_i) given $\mathbf{z}$ for the censored data. Therefore, for censored data, the alternative estimating equation is given by

$$\sum_{i=1}^{n} \Delta_i \mathbf{z}_i I(X_i > t_0)[\tau - I\{X_i \leq t_0 + \exp(\boldsymbol{\beta}'_{\tau|t_0}\mathbf{z}_i)\}] = 0. \quad (3.39)$$

Assuming independence between the censoring distribution and the covariates, i.e. with Δ_i unconditionally based on (X_i, δ_i), Kim *et al.* (2012) showed that the estimator for $\boldsymbol{\beta}_{\tau|t_0}$ from Eq. (3.39) is asymptotically consistent for the true parameter and follows an asymptotically normal distribution. The independence assumption is rather strong, but it often holds for a well-conducted clinical trial where the major cause of censoring is administrative. When the independence assumption is suspicious, a jump of the conditional cumulative probability, $F(X_i|\mathbf{z}_i)$, can be estimated from a stratified or adjusted Kaplan–Meier estimator (Xie and Liu, 2005). The function rq.wfit with the option of choosing the weights as Δ_i in the procedure WRegEst from the R package emplik can be modified to obtain the estimate of $\boldsymbol{\beta}_{\tau|t_0}$ from Eq. (3.39) (see Example 3.11).

Now let us consider testing the null hypothesis $H_0 : \boldsymbol{\beta}_{\tau|t_0} = \boldsymbol{\beta}_{\tau|t_0,0}$. As shown in Sect. 3.1, the variance of the quantile function, and hence the quantile residual life function, involves the probability density function of the underlying distribution. Similarly, because the limiting variance–covariance matrix of the estimators $\hat{\boldsymbol{\beta}}_{\tau|t_0}$ involves unknown conditional probability density functions of $\log(T_i - t_0) - \boldsymbol{\beta}'_{\tau|t_0,0}\mathbf{z}_i$ given $\mathbf{z}_i$ under the model (3.27), Jung *et al.* (2009) used the estimating function $\mathbf{S}_{t_0,n}(\boldsymbol{\beta}_{\tau|t_0})$ directly to test H_0. They showed that, by using the multivariate central limit theorem, the distribution of $n^{-1/2}\mathbf{S}_{\tau|t_0,n}(\boldsymbol{\beta}^0_{\tau|t_0})$ is asymptotically normal with mean 0 and a variance–covariance matrix, which can be consistently estimated by

$$\hat{\boldsymbol{\Gamma}}_{\tau|t_0}(\hat{\boldsymbol{\beta}}_{\tau|t_0}) = n^{-1}\sum_{i=1}^{n}\hat{\boldsymbol{\xi}}_{\tau|t_0,i}\hat{\boldsymbol{\xi}}'_{\tau|t_0,i}, \tag{3.40}$$

where

$$\hat{\boldsymbol{\xi}}_{\tau|t_0,i} = \left[\frac{I\{X_i > t_0 + \exp(\hat{\boldsymbol{\beta}}'_{\tau|t_0}\mathbf{z}_i)\}}{\hat{G}\{t_0 + \exp(\hat{\boldsymbol{\beta}}'_{\tau|t_0}\mathbf{z}_i)\}} - (1-\tau)\frac{I(X_i > t_0)}{\hat{G}(t_0)}\right]\mathbf{z}_i$$

$$+ \sum_{l=1}^{n}\left[\mathbf{z}_l\frac{I\{t_0 + \exp(\hat{\boldsymbol{\beta}}'_{\tau|t_0}\mathbf{z}_l) < X_l\}}{\hat{G}\{t_0 + \exp(\hat{\boldsymbol{\beta}}'_{\tau|t_0}\mathbf{z}_l)\}}\right]\left[\frac{(1-\delta_i)I\{X_i \le t_0 + \exp(\hat{\boldsymbol{\beta}}'_{\tau|t_0}\mathbf{z}_l)\}}{\sum_{m=1}^{n}I(X_m \ge X_i)}\right.$$

$$\left. - \sum_{j=1}^{n}\frac{(1-\delta_j)I[X_j \le \min\{t_0 + \exp(\hat{\boldsymbol{\beta}}'_{\tau|t_0}\mathbf{z}_l), X_i\}]}{\{\sum_{m=1}^{n}I(X_m \ge X_j)\}^2}\right]$$

$$- \sum_{l=1}^{n}\left\{\mathbf{z}_l\frac{(1-\tau)I(X_l > t_0)}{n\hat{G}(t_0)}\right\}\left[\frac{(1-\delta_i)I(X_i \le t_0)}{\sum_{m=1}^{n}I(X_m \ge X_i)}\right.$$

$$\left. - \sum_{j=1}^{n}\frac{(1-\delta_j)I\{X_j \le \min(t_0, X_i)\}}{\{\sum_{m=1}^{n}I(X_m \ge X_j)\}^2}\right],$$

where $\hat{\boldsymbol{\beta}}_{\tau|t_0}$ is a consistent estimate of the true parameter $\boldsymbol{\beta}^0_{\tau|t_0}$.

A natural test statistic based on $\mathbf{S}_{\tau|t_0,n}(\boldsymbol{\beta}_{\tau|t_0,0})$ for testing H_0 would be

$$n^{-1}\mathbf{S}'_{\tau|t_0,n}(\boldsymbol{\beta}_{\tau|t_0,0})\hat{\boldsymbol{\Gamma}}^{-1}_{\tau|t_0}(\hat{\boldsymbol{\beta}}_{\tau|t_0})\mathbf{S}_{\tau|t_0,n}(\boldsymbol{\beta}_{\tau|t_0,0}), \tag{3.41}$$

which approximately follows a χ^2-distribution with $p+1$ degrees of freedom. A large observed value of this statistic suggests evidence against the null hypothesis H_0. Jung *et al.* (2009) also showed that the distribution of $\hat{\boldsymbol{\beta}}_{\tau|t_0}$ is asymptotically normal for given $\mathbf{z}_i$ and fixed t_0 based on the local linearity of $\mathbf{S}_{\tau|t_0,n}(\boldsymbol{\beta}_{\tau|t_0})$.

Now let us consider a partition of the regression coefficients, $\boldsymbol{\beta}'_{\tau|t_0} = (\boldsymbol{\beta}^{(1)}_{\tau|t_0}{}', \boldsymbol{\beta}^{(2)}_{\tau|t_0}{}')$, where $\boldsymbol{\beta}^{(1)}_{\tau|t_0}$ is an $r \times 1$ vector. Suppose that $\hat{\boldsymbol{\beta}}^{(1)}_{\tau|t_0}$ and $\hat{\boldsymbol{\beta}}^{(2)}_{\tau|t_0}$ are the corresponding estimates, and we are only interested in testing the hypothesis $\tilde{H}_0 : \boldsymbol{\beta}^{(1)}_{\tau|t_0} = \boldsymbol{\beta}^{(1)}_{\tau|t_0,0}$, a specified vector, against a general alternative. Jung *et al.* (2009)

proposed a variation of the minimum dispersion statistic (Basawa and Koul, 1988),

$$V(\boldsymbol{\beta}_{\tau|t_0,0}^{(1)}) = \min_{\boldsymbol{\beta}_{\tau|t_0}^{(2)}} \{n^{-1}\mathbf{S}_{t_0,n}'((\boldsymbol{\beta}_{\tau|t_0,0}^{(1)}{}',\boldsymbol{\beta}_{\tau|t_0}^{(2)}{}'))$$
$$\times \hat{\boldsymbol{\Gamma}}_{\tau|t_0}^{-1}(\hat{\boldsymbol{\beta}}_{\tau|t_0})\mathbf{S}_{t_0,n}((\boldsymbol{\beta}_{\tau|t_0,0}^{(1)}{}',\boldsymbol{\beta}_{\tau|t_0}^{(2)}{}'))\}. \quad (3.42)$$

Note that evaluating this statistic does not require estimation of the probability density function of the survival distribution, which is needed for a Wald-type test statistic based on $\hat{\boldsymbol{\beta}}_{\tau|t_0}$. By using similar arguments given in Wei, Ying, and Lin (1990, Appendix 2) and Ying et al. (1995, Appendix C), it can be shown that (3.42) is approximately χ^2-distributed with r degrees of freedom (Jung et al., 2009). We reject $\tilde{H}_0$ for a large value of $V(\boldsymbol{\beta}_{\tau|t_0,0}^{(1)})$. By inverting this test statistic, a $100 \times (1-\alpha)\%$ confidence region for $\boldsymbol{\beta}_{\tau|t_0}^{(1)}$ can be obtained as

$$\{\boldsymbol{\beta}_{\tau|t_0}^{(1)} : V(\boldsymbol{\beta}_{\tau|t_0}^{(1)}) < \chi_{1-\alpha,r}^2\},$$

where $\chi_{1-\alpha,r}^2$ is the $100 \times (1-\alpha)^{th}$ percentile of a χ^2-distribution with r degrees of freedom.

Example 3.11. As introduced in Sect. 3.6, we consider a simple median residual life regression model

$$\text{median}\{\log(T_i - t_0)|T_i > t_0, z_{1i}\} = \beta_{t_0}^{(0)} + \beta_{t_0}^{(1)}z_{1i},$$

or equivalently

$$\text{median}(T_i - t_0|T_i > t_0, z_{1i}) = \exp(\beta_{t_0}^{(0)} + \beta_{t_0}^{(1)}z_{1i}),$$

where z_{1i} is a binary covariate, say, 0 for the control group and 1 for an intervention group. Under this model, recall that $\exp(\beta_{t_0}^{(0)})$ is the median residual lifetime at t_0 in the control group, or under the null hypothesis of $\tilde{H}_0 : \beta_{t_0}^{(1)} = 0$.

Suppose that failure times T_i follow a Weibull distribution with survival function $S(t) = \exp(-\lambda t^\kappa)$. For this distribution, note that under $\tilde{H}_0 : \beta_{t_0}^{(1)} = 0$, we have the median residual life-time at time t_0 as

$$
\begin{aligned}
\theta_{t_0} \equiv \exp(\beta_{t_0}^{(0)}) &= S^{-1}\{(1/2)S(t_0)\} - t_0 \\
&= \{\log(2)/\lambda_0 + t_0^\kappa\}^{1/\kappa} - t_0, \quad t_0 \geq 0. \quad (3.43)
\end{aligned}
$$

Note that by setting $\theta_{t_0} = \exp(\beta_{t_0}^{(0)})$ under $\tilde{H}_0$, we have $\lambda_0 = \{\log(2)\}/\exp(\beta_0^{(0)})^\kappa$ when $t_0 = 0$.

By using the probability integral transformation, failure times were generated for both groups from $T_i = \{-\log(1 - U_i)/\lambda_0\}^{1/\kappa}$, where U_i is from a uniform random variable between 0 and 1. Under $\tilde{H}_0 : \beta_{t_0}^{(1)} = 0$, Eq. (3.43) gives the true values of $\beta_{t_0}^{(0)}$ as 1.61, 1.41, 1.22, and 1.04 at $t_0 = 0, 1, 2, 3$, respectively. We assumed that $\kappa = 2$ and $\exp(\beta_0^{(0)}) = 5$, implying that the shape parameter κ does not change in the surviving population. The true value of $\beta_{t_0}^{(1)}$ must be 0 for all $t_0 \geq 0$ because an identical survival distribution was assumed for both groups. Censoring times C_i were generated from a uniform distribution between 0 and c, where constant c is for a certain censoring proportion. Finally the observed survival times X_i were determined as the minimum of T_i and C_i.

For the illustrative purpose, we simulate a dataset with a small sample size of 20 under the scenario described above. Table 3.5 displays the simulated dataset including observed survival time (x_i), event indicator (δ_i), and group indicator (z_i).

Because optimization and numerical evaluation of the score statistic and its variance are complicated in this case, we provide the R codes (R Development Core Team, 2008) in Appendix A.3. The function MMRRegEst is to estimate the regression parameters $\beta_{t_0}^{(0)}$ and $\beta_{t_0}^{(1)}$ from Eq. (3.39). When $t_0 = 0$, the estimates were 1.64 and -0.42, respectively, which are slightly off the targets due to the small sample size. With an increase of the sample size to 500 gave more accurate estimates of 1.60 and -0.01. With the small sample estimates plugged in, the estimated variance–covariance matrix for the score functions in (3.40) was

$$
\hat{\Gamma}_{\tau|t_0}(\hat{\beta}_{\tau|t_0}) = \begin{pmatrix} 0.2743 & 0.1371 \\ 0.1371 & 0.1508 \end{pmatrix},
$$

Table 3.5: A simulated dataset from a Weibull distribution: x_i, observed survival time; $\delta_i=1$ for event and 0 for censored; $z_i=0$ for control group and 1 for intervention group

x_i, observed survival time	δ_i, event indicator	z_i, group indicator
0.586	1	1
0.818	1	1
1.077	1	0
1.533	0	1
1.766	1	0
1.775	0	0
2.390	1	0
3.053	1	1
3.374	1	1
3.387	1	1
3.438	1	1
4.774	1	0
5.166	1	0
6.089	1	0
6.317	1	0
6.798	1	0
7.076	1	1
7.174	1	1
9.642	1	0
12.950	1	1

so that the statistic for the global test of the null hypothesis H_0 : $\boldsymbol{\beta}_{\tau|t_0,0} = (\beta_{t_0}^{(0)}, \beta_{t_0}^{(1)}) = (0,0)$ in (3.41) was estimated as

$$n^{-1}\mathbf{S}'_{\tau|t_0,n}(\boldsymbol{\beta}_{\tau|t_0,0})\hat{\boldsymbol{\Gamma}}^{-1}_{\tau|t_0}(\hat{\boldsymbol{\beta}}_{\tau|t_0})\mathbf{S}_{\tau|t_0,n}(\boldsymbol{\beta}_{\tau|t_0,0}) = 12.27,$$

which is greater than $\chi^2_{0.95,2} = 5.99$, implying that at least one of the regression parameters deviates significantly from 0 at the significance level of 0.05.

Now to perform the local test of the null hypothesis $\tilde{H}_0 : \beta_{t_0}^{(1)} = 0$, the grid search method was used to estimate the minimum dispersion statistic in (3.42). The estimate was

$$V(0) = \min_{\beta_{t_0}^{(0)}}\{n^{-1}\mathbf{S}'_{t_0,n}((\beta_{t_0}^{(0)},0))\hat{\mathbf{\Gamma}}_{\tau|t_0}^{-1}(\hat{\boldsymbol{\beta}}_{\tau|t_0})\mathbf{S}_{t_0,n}((\beta_{t_0}^{(0)},0))\} = 0.95,$$

which is smaller than $\chi^2_{0.95,1} = 3.84$, implying that the slope coefficient is not significantly different from 0 at the significance level of 0.05. Together with the result from the global test, this also implies that the intercept, or the logarithm of the median residual lifetime in the control group, is significantly greater than 0 at the significance level of 0.05.

Example 3.12 (Application to NSABP B-04 Data). Jung *et al.* (2009) applied the regression analysis based on the estimating equation (3.37) and the variance formula (3.42) to the NSABP B-04 dataset. They have included age at surgery (*age*), nodal status (*node*) (negative or positive), and tumor size (*tsize*) as covariates in the regression model (3.27). Age and tumor size values were rescaled by being multiplied by 0.01, so that the regularity condition holds in the estimates of the censoring distribution in the estimating equation. Table 3.6 summarizes the analysis results from Jung *et al.* (2009).

The results show that all the covariate effects are negative on the median residual lifetimes at any fixed time points. Specifically, the negative effect of age at diagnosis tends to get worse at later time points, whereas the effects of nodal status and pathological tumor size are significant only through first 4 or 5 years, when adjusting for other cov ariates. These results can be used to predict a patient's median residual lifetime at a given time t_0 as baseline information without adjuvant chemo- or hormonal therapies, as pointed out by Jung *et al.* (2009). For example, for a patient with positive lymph nodes, median age at diagnosis of 56, and median pathological tumor size of 30 mm, the median residual lifetime 6 years after the original diagnosis of cancer was predicted as $\exp\{3.92-1\times0.28-2.11\times(0.01\times56.0)-0.48\times(0.01\times30.0)\} = 10.1$. For node-negative patients, similarly, the predicted median residual lifetime was 13.4 years.

Table 3.6: Regression parameter estimates from the median residual life regression model with multiple covariates and 95% confidence intervals (CI) for testing the null hypothesis $H_0 : \beta_i = 0$ ($i = 0$, *intercept*; $i = 1$, *node*; $i = 2$, *age*; $i = 3$, *tsize*) [Jung *et al.*, 2009, *Biometrics*]

t_0	$\hat{\beta}_0$	95% CI	$\hat{\beta}_1$	95% CI	$\hat{\beta}_2$	95% CI	$\hat{\beta}_3$	95% CI
0	3.29	(2.91,4.24)	−.51	(−.72,−.32)	−.83	(−2.33,−.21)	−1.02	(−1.85,−.61)
2	3.94	(3.31,4.83)	−.44	(−.65,−.21)	−2.06	(−3.17,−1.10)	−.89	(−1.18,−.40)
4	4.06	(3.43,4.79)	−.35	(−.63,−.13)	−2.29	(−3.38,−1.63)	−.71	(−1.59,.97)
6	3.92	(3.54,4.68)	−.14	(−.65,.10)	−2.11	(−3.65,−1.59)	−.48	(−1.40,.96)
8	3.88	(3.42,4.77)	−1.60	(−.51,.13)	−2.21	(−3.18,−1.61)	−.36	(−1.05,.81)
10	3.87	(3.27,4.84)	−.10	(−.47,.12)	−2.33	(−3.90,−1.60)	−.36	(−.91,.84)

3.7 Further Reading and Future Direction

A general concept of the τ-quantile residual life function was originally introduced by Haines and Singpurwalla (1974). One of the major difficulties in making inferences based on the quantile residual function is a non-uniqueness of the corresponding life distribution. This problem has been intensively explored by many authors (Schmittlein and Morrison, 1981; Arnold and Brockett, 1983; Joe and Proschan, 1984; Joe, 1985; Song and Cho, 1995 and Lillo, 2005). Gupta and Langford (1984) under mild assumptions determined a general form of distribution when its median residual life function is known. Ghosh and Mustafi (1986), Csörgö and Csörgö (1987), and Alam and Kulasekera (1993), among others, investigated asymptotic properties of the sample quantile residual life process. Also substantial amount of work was done on the confidence bands for the quantile residual life function (Barabas *et al.*, 1986; Aly, 1992; Chung, 1989; Csörgö and Viharos, 1992). Recently, Franco-Pereira *et al.* (2012) proposed a nonparametric method for constructing confidence bands for the difference of the two quantile residual life functions based on the functional depth (López-Pintado and Romo, 2009). Bandos (2007) proposed a proportional scaled quantile residual life model, but the interpretation of the regression parameters in terms of the quantile residual life functions is not clear, as in the proportional scaled mean residual life model (Liu and Ghosh, 2008). Ma and Yin (2009) proposed a general class of the semiparametric median residual life regression model and formulated the estimating equation via the "check" function, which can be shown to be equivalent to Eq. (3.39) because the jumps of the Kaplan–Meier estimator are closely related to the inversely weighted censoring probability (see Sect. 5.2.2). Ma and Wei (2012) considered estimation of the time-varying coefficients for the quantile residual life regression model.

Interestingly, Kim and Yang (2011) extended the quantile regression model to a clustered response data without censoring, by using the empirical likelihood and Markov chain and Monte carlo (MCMC) samplers in the Bayesian framework. Their results presented in this chapter might be able to be further extended to the quantile residual life model with random effects. A length-biased sample arises in survival data when investigators are interested in estimating the quantile residual lifetime to death, for example, among patients who recurred *within* 5 years after the initial treatment. Extension might be useful for this case as well.

Chapter 4

Quantile Residual Life Under Competing Risks

Competing risks data are often encountered in many research areas such as medicine, engineering, and econometrics whenever one type of events precludes other types of events from being observed. For example, in cancer research, investigators might want to know a drug effect that would only affect a disease-specific endpoint, say time-to-death due to breast cancer. In this case, any death due to other causes that occurs first would preclude a breast-cancer-related death from being observed. In this chapter, we extend the results developed in Chap. 3 to both parametric and nonparametric competing risks settings. We first review statistical literature on competing risks. Then we define the cumulative distribution function for the residual life distribution under competing risks, an inversion of which would provide the quantile residual lifetime for a subdistribution of a specific event type. For parametric inference on two-sample case and parametric regression, we extend existing methods to infer the quantile residual life under competing risks by using the maximum likelihood principle. For nonparametric inference on one-sample and two-sample cases and semiparametric inference, we review recent work by Jeong and Fine (2009, 2013) and Lim (2011). R codes used in the numerical examples are provided in Appendix.

J.-H. Jeong, *Statistical Inference on Residual Life,*
Statistics for Biology and Health, DOI 10.1007/978-1-4939-0005-3_4,
© Springer Science+Business Media New York 2014

4.1   Competing Risks

The history of the concept of competing risks dates back to the eighteenth century when Daniel Bernoulli attempted to adjust the survival probability from the life tables developed by Edmond Halley after eliminating smallpox as a cause of death (David and Moeschberger, 1978; Pintilie, 2006). In this section, we review the fundamental quantities that are commonly used in the analysis of competing risks data, such as cause-specific hazard, subdistribution hazard, and the cumulative incidence function.

4.1.1   Cause-Specific Hazard and Cumulative Incidence Function

When investigators are interested in estimating the cumulative probability of the cause-specific events of interest in the presence of competing events, one potentially tempting approach would be to censor the competing events at the time of occurrence, and calculate the complement of the Kaplan–Meier estimator (Kaplan and Meier, 1958), which will be referred to as 1-KM. However, it is well known that the 1-KM approach overestimates the true *cumulative* probability of the cause-specific events (Korn and Dorey, 1992; Pepe and Mori, 1993; Gaynor, Feuer et al., 1993; Lin, 1997). The cumulative incidence function (Kalbfleisch and Prentice, 1980) provides the correct estimate for the cumulative probability of the cause-specific events in the presence of competing events without assumptions about the dependence among the risks.

The basic identifiable quantities from competing risks data (T, ϵ) are the cause-specific hazard and cumulative incidence functions, where T is time to the first event under competing risks with an index $\epsilon = 1, 2, \ldots, J$ for a set of mutually exclusive competing events. We first derive the cumulative incidence function from the cause-specific hazard function. The cause-specific hazard function is the limiting conditional probability that an individual would experience an event $\epsilon = j$ at time t given that he/she did not have any event up to t, that is,

$$h_j(t) = \lim_{\Delta \to 0} \frac{\Pr(t \le T < t + \Delta, \epsilon = j | T \ge t)}{\Delta}.$$

We see that, for a small Δ,

$$
\begin{aligned}
h_j(t)\Delta &\approx \Pr(t \le T < t + \Delta, \epsilon = j | T \ge t) \\
&= \Pr(t \le T < t + \Delta, \epsilon = j)/\Pr(T \ge t),
\end{aligned}
$$

which implies

$$\Pr(t \le T < t + \Delta, \epsilon = j) \approx \Pr(T \ge t)h_j(t)\Delta. \tag{4.1}$$

Noticing that the left-hand side in (4.1) approximates the probability density function for the type j events, say $f_j(t)$, as $\Delta \to 0$, the cumulative probability of the type j events can be obtained by integrating both sides in (4.1) as $\Delta \to 0$. Thus the cumulative incidence function for the type j events can be defined as

$$F_j(t) \equiv \Pr(T \le t, \epsilon = j) = \int_0^t f_j(u)du = \int_0^t S(u-)d\Lambda_j(u), \tag{4.2}$$

where $S(t) = \Pr(T > t)$ and $\Lambda_j(t) = \int_0^t h_j(u)du$ is the cumulative hazard function for the type j events. We can easily see that the cumulative incidence function is improper because

$$
\begin{aligned}
\lim_{t \to \infty} F_j(t) &= \lim_{t \to \infty} \Pr(T \le t, \epsilon = j) \\
&= \lim_{t \to \infty} \Pr(T \le t | \epsilon = j)\Pr(\epsilon = j) = \Pr(\epsilon = j),
\end{aligned}
$$

so that the empirical version of the cumulative incidence function for a random sample of $T_1, T_2, \ldots, T_n$ can be expressed as

$$\hat{F}_j^*(t) = \frac{1}{n} \sum_{i=1}^{n} I(T_i \le t, \epsilon = j). \tag{4.3}$$

Parametrically, the cumulative incidence function $F_j(t)$ can be directly modeled by a family of improper distributions such as Gompertz (Jeong and Fine, 2006). For nonparametric estimation of the cumulative incidence function in Eq. (4.2), the overall survival function $S(\cdot)$ may be replaced by the Kaplan–Meier estimator, and the cause-specific cumulative hazard function $\Lambda_j(\cdot)$ may be replaced by a Nelson–Aalen estimator (Nelson, 1972; Aalen, 1978) after treating the competing events as independent censoring. This leads to the nonparametric estimator of the cumulative incidence function for type j events as

$$\hat{F}_j(t) = \sum_{t_i \leq t} \left\{ \prod_{k=1}^{i-1} \left(1 - \frac{d_k + r_k}{Y_k} \right) \right\} \left(\frac{r_i}{Y_i} \right), \tag{4.4}$$

where Y_k is the number of subjects at risk at an ordered observed event time t_k, and r_k and d_k are numbers of type j events and the other events at time t_k, respectively.

4.1.2   Subdistribution Hazard Function

For the right-censored data, let us denote $X = \min(T, C)$ for the independent censoring time C and $\delta = I(T \leq C)$ is the event indicator function. Another nonparametric approach to modeling the cumulative incidence function would be to introduce the improper random variable (Gray, 1988; Fine and Gray, 1999), ignoring the fact that competing events have occurred, so that they are not censored at the time of occurrence. When there is no censoring, the improper random variable is defined as

$$T^* = I(\epsilon = j) \times T + \{1 - I(\epsilon = j)\} \times \infty,$$

so that the subdistribution hazard function is

$$\begin{aligned} \gamma_j(t) &= \lim_{\Delta \to 0} \frac{\Pr(t \leq T < t + \Delta, \epsilon = j | T \geq t \cup (T \leq t \cap \epsilon \neq j)}{\Delta} \\ &= \frac{f_j(t)}{1 - F_j(t)} = -\frac{d}{dt} \log\{1 - F_j(t)\}. \end{aligned} \tag{4.5}$$

Note that hypothetically all the subjects who had competing events would be included indefinitely in the risk set in (4.5). For the competing events considered as dependently censored, the risk indicator for the event type j would be unknown thereafter, making the usual counting and risk processes incomputable. To estimate the potential times for the competing events to remain in the risk set, Fine and Gray (1999) extended the inverse probability censoring weighting (IPCW) by noticing that multiplying the risk indicator for the event type j into the usual risk and counting processes make them still computable. Specifically the weight function for the ith individual at time t is given by

$$w_i(t) = \frac{r_i(t)\hat{G}(t)}{\hat{G}(\min(X_i, t))},$$

where $X_i = \min(T_i, C_i)$, $r_i(t) = I(X_i \geq t \cup (\delta_i = 1 \cap \epsilon_i \neq j))$ is the risk indicator function for the event type j, ignoring occurrence of the competing events, and $\hat{G}(\cdot)$ is the Kaplan–Meier estimator based on $\{(X_i, 1 - \delta_i), i = 1, 2, \ldots, n\}$. As further clarified by Katsahian *et al.* (2006), the weight would stay as 1 only until a type j event or a right censoring occurs, and then drop to 0. After a competing event occurs, however, the weight would be decreasing over time.

There exists an interesting relationship between the cause-specific hazard function and the subdistribution hazard function as shown in Beyersmann *et al.* (2007, 2009). From Eqs. (4.2) and (4.5), we have

$$f_j(t) = S(t)h_j(t) = \gamma_j(t)\{1 - F_j(t)\},$$

which gives

$$h_j(t) = \left\{\frac{1 - F_j(t)}{S(t)}\right\}\gamma_j(t).$$

This implies that when there are no competing events, the cause-specific hazard and subdistribution hazard functions become identical, but the cause-specific hazard is always higher than the subdistribution hazard under competing risks because $S(t) \leq 1 - F_j(t)$.

4.1.3 Bivariate Point of View

The cumulative incidence function can also be derived from a bivariate point of view. Let us define $T = \min(T_1, T_2)$ without censoring, implying that T would be the time to event that occurs first when two types of events are competing. As a specific example, let us consider Fig. 4.1 where the bivariate probabilities are defined on the grid support points between 1 and 5 for both T_1 and T_2. One can see that the probability of $T = 3$ can be expressed as

$$P(T = 3) = \sum_{i=3}^{5} \{P(T_1 = i, T_2 = 3) + P(T_2 = i, T_1 = 3)\}$$
$$- P(T_1 = 3, T_2 = 3),$$

so in general we can write

$$P(T=t) = P(T_1 \geq t, T_2=t) + P(T_2 \geq t, T_1=t) - P(T_1=t, T_2=t)$$
$$= P(T \geq t) \{h_2(t) + h_1(t) - h_{12}(t)\}, \qquad (4.6)$$

where, for $j = 1, 2$,

$$h_j(t) = \frac{-(\partial/\partial t_j)P(T_1 \geq t_1, T_2 \geq t_2)|_{t_1=t_2=t}}{P(T \geq t)}$$

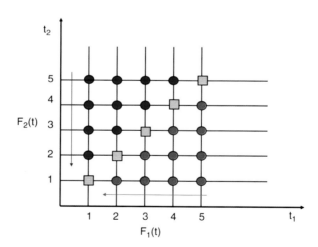

Fig. 4.1: Defining the cumulative incidence function in the bivariate setting

is the cause-specific hazard function for type j events and

$$h_{12}(t) = \frac{\frac{\partial^2}{\partial t_1 \partial t_2}P(T_1 \geq t_1, T_2 \geq t_2)|_{t_1=t_2=t}}{P(T \geq t)}$$

is the joint hazard function.

Because only the event that occurs first is observed under competing risks, from (4.6) the probability density function for a cause-specific type j $(j = 1, 2)$ event is given by

$$P(T = t, j = 1) = P(T_2 \geq t, T_1 = t) = P(T \geq t)h_1(t),$$

and

$$P(T = t, j = 2) = P(T_1 \geq t, T_2 = t) = P(T \geq t)h_2(t),$$

respectively. Integrating both sides in the above equations leads to the definition of the cumulative incidence function for each type events. Therefore in Fig. 4.1, the subdistribution of type 1 events is defined as the vertical sums of the probabilities assigned to the grids in the upper triangular area and the subdistribution of type 2 events is defined as the horizontal sums of the probabilities assigned to the grids in the lower triangular area. The probabilities assigned to the diagonal grids are often assumed to be 0 for practical convenience.

4.2 Quantile Residual Life Under Competing Risks

As mentioned in the previous section, investigators might be often interested in cause-specific treatment effects in terms of extending a patient's remaining life years, e.g. the median residual lifetime to a breast-cancer-related-death. In this section, we define the quantile for the residual life distribution under competing risks.

First, the importance of using the correct method under competing risks can be further emphasized when the quantile residual life function is concerned. Figure 4.2 (Jeong and Fine, 2013) shows the estimated cumulative probability of breast-cancer-related deaths from a subset of a phase III clinical trial dataset by using the 1-KM method and the cumulative incidence function for the residual life distributions at follow-up years of 0, 1, 2, and 3, respectively. The median residual life years can be estimated by inverting the estimated curves in each panel (see the dotted lines).

One can notice that the gap between the two median residual life estimates widens as the fixed follow-up year increases. For example, the difference between the two estimates at follow-up year 3 is about 10 years (24.4 vs. 14.6). This warns that the 1-KM approach should be avoided especially in estimating the quantiles of the cause-specific residual life distribution.

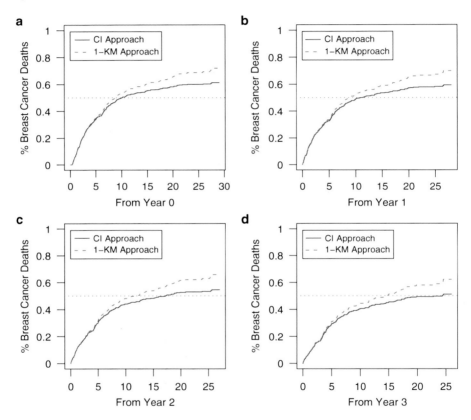

Fig. 4.2: Comparison between two approaches to estimating quantile residual lifetimes under competing risks; 1-KM vs. Cumulative Incidence Function (Jeong and Fine, 2013, *Biometrical Journal*)

Let us now define the cumulative distribution function for the residual life distribution at a fixed time t_0 in terms of the all-cause survival function $S(t)$ as

$$F_{t_0}(t) = \mathrm{P}(T - t_0 \leq t | T > t_0) = \{S(t_0) - S(t + t_0)\}/S(t_0).$$

Similarly, for a specific cause j under competing risks, Jeong and Fine (2009) defined the cumulative incidence function for the residual life distribution given survival up to t_0 as

$$
\begin{aligned}
F_{j,t_0}(t) &= \mathrm{P}(T - t_0 \leq t, \epsilon = j | T > t_0) \\
&= \{F_j(t + t_0) - F_j(t_0)\}/S(t_0), \quad (4.7)
\end{aligned}
$$

where $F_j(\cdot)$ is the cumulative incidence function for type j events. Therefore the τ-quantile residual life estimator of cause j, $\hat{\theta}_{j,t_0}(\tau)$, can be estimated from the equation

$$
u\{\theta_{j,t_0}(\tau)\} = \hat{F}_j\{t_0 + \theta_{j,t_0}(\tau)\} - \hat{F}_j(t_0) - \tau \hat{S}(t_0) = 0, \quad (4.8)
$$

where $\hat{F}_j(\cdot)$ and $\hat{S}(\cdot)$ are parametric or nonparametric estimators of the cumulative incidence function for type j events, $F_j(\cdot)$, and all-cause survival function, $S(\cdot)$, respectively.

4.3 Parametric Inference

In this section, we present the parametric inference methods for the quantiles for the residual life distribution of events of interest under competing risks. As long as the observed data fit a parametric distribution reasonably well, a parametric inference would provide more accurate analysis results. Another advantage of the parametric inference particularly on the quantiles would be no need to use a smoothing method for estimation of the probability density function under competing risks to evaluate the variance of the quantile estimate.

4.3.1 One-Sample Case

For notational simplicity, suppose there are only two types of competing events, type 1 and type 2, with type 1 events being of interest. Jeong and Fine (2006) compared two parameterization methods for the cumulative incidence function; direct vs. cause-specific. First we consider inference on the τ-quantile residual life function through the direct parameterization.

Direct Parameterization

The direct parameterization assumes the additivity of two cause-specific cumulative incidence functions, i.e. $F(t) = F_1(t) + F_2(t)$, where $F(t)$ is the all-cause cumulative distribution function and $F_j(t)$ $(j = 1, 2)$ is the cumulative incidence function for type j events. Therefore, with smooth cumulative incidence functions of $F_1(\cdot; \boldsymbol{\psi}_1)$ and $F_2(\cdot; \boldsymbol{\psi}_2)$ with parameter vectors $\boldsymbol{\psi}_1$ and $\boldsymbol{\psi}_2$, the direct parameterization would give $S(\cdot; \boldsymbol{\psi}) = 1 - F_1(\cdot; \boldsymbol{\psi}_1) - F_2(\cdot; \boldsymbol{\psi}_2)$, where $\boldsymbol{\psi} = (\boldsymbol{\psi}_1^T, \boldsymbol{\psi}_2^T)^T$.

Thus, the τ-quantile for the residual life distribution of type 1 events from (4.8) is given by

$$\theta_{1,t_0}(\tau; \boldsymbol{\psi}) = F_1^{-1}[F_1(t_0; \boldsymbol{\psi}_1) + \tau\{1 - F_1(t_0; \boldsymbol{\psi}_1) - F_2(t_0; \boldsymbol{\psi}_2)\}; \boldsymbol{\psi}_1] - t_0. \tag{4.9}$$

Once the invertible cumulative incidence functions are specified, a parametric form of the residual life τ-quantile can be analytically expressed.

To estimate $\theta_{1,t_0}(\tau; \boldsymbol{\psi})$, we first need to estimate the parameter vectors $\boldsymbol{\psi}_1$ and $\boldsymbol{\psi}_2$ from the maximum the likelihood function under competing risks, which is generally given by

$$L(\boldsymbol{\psi}) = \prod_{i=1}^{n} f_1(x_i; \boldsymbol{\psi}_1)^{\delta_{1i}} f_2(x_i; \boldsymbol{\psi}_2)^{\delta_{2i}} S(x_i; \boldsymbol{\psi})^{1-\delta_{1i}-\delta_{2i}}, \tag{4.10}$$

where

$$f_j(x; \boldsymbol{\psi}_j) = dF_j(x; \boldsymbol{\psi}_j)/dx, \quad j = 1, 2 \tag{4.11}$$

is an improper probability density function for the distribution of type j events, $S(x_i; \boldsymbol{\psi})$ is the all-cause survival function, and δ_{ji} is the indicator function for a type j event, i.e. $\delta_{ji} = 1$ if the ith subject experiences an event type j and 0 otherwise. Under the direct parameterization, the likelihood function (4.10) can be rewritten as (Jeong and Fine, 2006)

$$\prod_{i=1}^{n} f_1(x_i; \boldsymbol{\psi}_1)^{\delta_{1i}} f_2(x_i; \boldsymbol{\psi}_2)^{\delta_{2i}} \{1 - F_1(x_i; \boldsymbol{\psi}_1) - F_2(x_i; \boldsymbol{\psi}_2)\}^{1-\delta_{1i}-\delta_{2i}}.$$

$$\tag{4.12}$$

Example 4.1 (Gompertz Distribution). Let us consider the two-parameter Gompertz distribution for the cumulative incidence function for type j events at $t_0 = 0$, that is

$$F_j(x; \boldsymbol{\psi}_j) = 1 - \exp[\kappa_j\{1 - \exp(\rho_j x)\}/\rho_j], \qquad (4.13)$$

where $\boldsymbol{\psi}_j = (\rho_j, \kappa_j)$ $(j = 1, 2)$. Note that when $\rho_j < 0$, the cumulative incidence function $F_j(x; \boldsymbol{\psi}_j)$ has an improper asymptote $1 - \exp(\kappa_j/\rho_j)$ as $x \to \infty$. The likelihood function (4.12) would involve four parameters, two for each event type, which are estimated simultaneously. Now the estimates of $\boldsymbol{\psi}_1$ and $\boldsymbol{\psi}_2$, denoted as $\hat{\boldsymbol{\psi}}_1$ and $\hat{\boldsymbol{\psi}}_2$, can be plugged into (4.13) to estimate the cumulative incidence function for each cause, denoted as $F_1(t_0; \hat{\boldsymbol{\psi}}_1)$ and $F_2(t_0; \hat{\boldsymbol{\psi}}_2)$, and hence to estimate the τ-quantile residual life for type 1 events as

$$\theta_{1,t_0}(\tau; \hat{\boldsymbol{\psi}}) = F_1^{-1}[F_1(t_0; \hat{\boldsymbol{\psi}}_1) + \tau\{1 - F_1(t_0; \hat{\boldsymbol{\psi}}_1) - F_2(t_0; \hat{\boldsymbol{\psi}}_2)\}; \hat{\boldsymbol{\psi}}_1] - t_0.$$

By the invariance property of the maximum likelihood estimator, this estimator will be asymptotically consistent and normally distributed.

To find the variance of the τ-quantile residual life estimator $\theta_{1,t_0}(\tau; \hat{\boldsymbol{\psi}})$, we need to first obtain the observed information matrix for the parameter vector $\boldsymbol{\psi} = (\boldsymbol{\psi}_1^T, \boldsymbol{\psi}_2^T)^T = (\alpha_1, \beta_1, \alpha_2, \beta_2)$ by evaluating the negative second derivatives of the logarithm of the likelihood (4.12). Let us denote the 4×4 observed information matrix by $I_{(obs)}(\boldsymbol{\psi})$, so that the variance–covariance matrix is given by $I_{(obs)}^{-1}(\boldsymbol{\psi})$. Then, by applying the multivariate delta method, the asymptotic variance of the residual life cumulative incidence function for type 1 events at time t_0 can be evaluated by

$$\mathrm{Var}\left[F_{1,t_0}(x; \hat{\boldsymbol{\psi}})\right] = \left(\frac{\partial F_{1,t_0}(x; \boldsymbol{\psi})}{\partial \boldsymbol{\psi}}\right)^T I_{(obs)}^{-1}(\boldsymbol{\psi})\left(\frac{\partial F_{1,t_0}(x; \boldsymbol{\psi})}{\partial \boldsymbol{\psi}}\right),$$

where $\partial F_{1,t_0}(x; \boldsymbol{\psi})/\partial \boldsymbol{\psi}$ is a 4×1 vector containing the first derivatives of the residual life cumulative incidence function $F_{1,t_0}(x; \boldsymbol{\psi})$ with respect to the parameter vector $(\alpha_1, \beta_1, \alpha_2, \beta_2)$. This variance formula can be consistently estimated by replacing $\boldsymbol{\psi}$ with the maximum likelihood estimates $\hat{\psi}$. Applying the delta method once again, the variance of the τ-quantile residual life estimate for type 1 events at time t_0 under competing risks can be approximated by

$$\text{Var}\left[\theta_{1,t_0}(\tau;\hat{\psi})\right] = \frac{\text{Var}\left[F_{1,t_0}(\theta_{1,t_0}(\tau;\psi);\hat{\psi})\right]}{\{f_{1,t_0}(\theta_{1,t_0}(\tau;\psi);\psi)\}^2}, \tag{4.14}$$

where $f_{1,t_0}(t;\psi) = dF_{1,t_0}(t;\psi)/dt$, which can be specified from (4.7) as

$$f_{1,t_0}(t;\psi) = \frac{f_1(t+t_0;\psi_1)}{1 - F_1(t_0;\psi_1) - F_2(t_0;\psi_2)}.$$

Again the asymptotic variance of $\theta_{1,t_0}(\tau;\hat{\psi})$ can be consistently estimated by replacing ψ, $\theta_{1,t_0}(\tau;\psi)$, and $f_{1,t_0}(\theta_{1,t_0}(\tau;\psi);\psi)$ with the maximum likelihood estimates $\hat{\psi}$, $\theta_{1,t_0}(\tau;\hat{\psi})$, and $f_{1,t_0}(\theta_{1,t_0}(\tau;\hat{\psi});\hat{\psi})$.

Cause-Specific Parameterization

Under the cause-specific parameterization, the additive hazard property between two types of competing events leads to the multiplicity of two cause-specific pseudo-survival functions. That is, by denoting $h(t)$ is the all-cause hazard function and $h_j(t)$ $(j = 1, 2)$ is the cause-specific hazard function for type j events, the cause-specific parameterization assumes that $h(t) = h_1(t) + h_2(t)$, which implies that $S_1(t)S_2(t)$, where $S_j(t)$ $(j = 1, 2)$ is the pseudo-survival function for type j events. Together with the definition of $f_j(x;\psi)$ given in (4.11), under the cause-specific parameterization, the likelihood function (4.10) can be expressed as (Jeong and Fine, 2006)

$$\begin{aligned}
L(\psi) &= \prod_{i=1}^{n} f_1(x_i;\psi_1)^{\delta_{1i}} f_2(x_i;\psi_2)^{\delta_{2i}} S(x_i;\psi)^{1-\delta_{1i}-\delta_{2i}} \\
&= \prod_{i=1}^{n} \{S(x_i;\psi)h_1(x_i;\psi_1)\}^{\delta_{1i}} \{S(x_i;\psi)h_2(x_i;\psi_2)\}^{\delta_{2i}} \\
&\quad \times S(x_i;\psi)^{1-\delta_{1i}-\delta_{2i}}
\end{aligned}$$

$$= \prod_{i=1}^{n} h_1(x_i, \boldsymbol{\psi}_1)^{\delta_{1i}} h_2(x_i, \boldsymbol{\psi}_2)^{\delta_{2i}} \{S_1(x_i, \boldsymbol{\psi}_1) S_2(x_i, \boldsymbol{\psi}_2)\}.$$

$$(4.15)$$

Unlike the direct approach, the cause-specific hazard and all-cause survival functions in (4.15) can be modeled by the *proper* distributions (Prentice *et al.*, 1978; Jeong and Fine, 2006). As Jeong and Fine (2006) pointed out, the likelihood function (4.12) involves information from all event types and does not factor into separate pieces for each type. This differs from the parameterization based on the cause-specific hazard functions (Prentice *et al.*, 1978), where the likelihood function factors, so that inference about type 1 events of interest may be carried out separately from the models for type 2 events. Under the cause-specific hazard formulation, misspecification of cause-specific hazard functions for type 2 events does not lead to bias in the estimated model for type 1 events. However, a limitation of the cause-specific approach is that direct inference on the cumulative incidence functions is not possible.

As mentioned previously, one can easily see that the score function from the likelihood function (4.15) would have a simpler form than one under the direct parameterization. Taking the logarithm of (4.15) gives

$$l(\boldsymbol{\psi}) = \sum_{i=1}^{n} [\delta_{1i} \log\{h_1(x_i, \boldsymbol{\psi}_1)\} + \delta_{2i} \log\{h_2(x_i, \boldsymbol{\psi}_2)\}$$
$$+ \log\{S_1(x_i, \boldsymbol{\psi}_1)\} + \log\{S_2(x_i, \boldsymbol{\psi}_2)\}],$$

which has the first derivative with respect to $\boldsymbol{\psi}_1$ as

$$\frac{\partial l(\boldsymbol{\psi})}{\partial \boldsymbol{\psi}_1} = \sum_{i=1}^{n} \left\{ \delta_{i1} \frac{\partial h_1(x_i, \boldsymbol{\psi}_1)/\partial \boldsymbol{\psi}_1}{h_1(x_i, \boldsymbol{\psi}_1)} + \frac{\partial S_1(x_i, \boldsymbol{\psi}_1)/\partial \boldsymbol{\psi}_1}{S_1(x_i, \boldsymbol{\psi}_1)} \right\}. \quad (4.16)$$

Example 4.2 (Exponential Distribution). To obtain a closed form of the analytic results, suppose the cause-specific distribution for type 1 events follows an exponential with a rate parameter λ_1, so that the cause-specific hazard and survival function are given by $h_1(x, \lambda_1) = \lambda_1$ and $S_1(x, \lambda_1) = \exp(-\lambda_1 t)$, respectively. Then the score function in (4.16) simplifies to

$$\frac{\partial l(\lambda_1)}{\partial \lambda_1} = \sum_{i=1}^{n} \left(\frac{\delta_{1i}}{\lambda_1} - x_i \right). \qquad (4.17)$$

Setting the score function (4.17) to 0 and solving it for λ_1 gives the maximum likelihood estimator of λ_1 as

$$\hat{\lambda}_1 = \frac{\sum_{i=1}^{n} \delta_{1i}}{\sum_{i=1}^{n} x_i}.$$

The observed information can be obtained from the negative second derivative of the log-likelihood function as

$$I_{(obs)}(\lambda_1) = \frac{\partial^2 l(\lambda_1)}{\partial \lambda_1^2} = \frac{\sum_{i=1}^{n} \delta_{1i}}{\lambda_1^2},$$

so that the variance of $\hat{\lambda}_1$ can be consistently estimated by

$$\widehat{\mathrm{Var}}(\hat{\lambda}_1) = I_{(obs)}^{-1}(\hat{\lambda}_1) = \frac{\hat{\lambda}_1^2}{\sum_{i=1}^{n} \delta_{1i}} = \frac{\sum_{i=1}^{n} \delta_{1i}}{(\sum_{i=1}^{n} x_i)^2}.$$

Similarly, for the cause-specific distribution of type 2 events, we find

$$\hat{\lambda}_2 = \frac{\sum_{i=1}^{n} \delta_{2i}}{\sum_{i=1}^{n} x_i},$$

and

$$\widehat{\mathrm{Var}}(\hat{\lambda}_2) = \frac{\hat{\lambda}_2^2}{\sum_{i=1}^{n} \delta_{2i}} = \frac{\sum_{i=1}^{n} \delta_{2i}}{(\sum_{i=1}^{n} x_i)^2}.$$

Under the cause-specific parameterization via the exponential distribution, the τ-quantile for the residual life distribution of type 1 events is defined as

$$\theta_{1,t_0}^{(CS)}(\tau; \boldsymbol{\psi}) = F_1^{-1}[F_1(t_0; \lambda_1) + \tau S_1(t_0; \lambda_1)S_2(t_0; \lambda_2); \lambda_1] - t_0, \qquad (4.18)$$

where $\boldsymbol{\psi} = (\lambda_1, \lambda_2)$. Because $F_1^{-1}(v) = -(1/\lambda_1)\log(1 - v)$, Eq. (4.18) simplifies to

$$\theta_{1,t_0}^{(CS)}(\tau; \boldsymbol{\psi}) = -\frac{1}{\lambda_1} \log \left(1 - \tau e^{-\lambda_2 t_0} \right), \qquad (4.19)$$

which can be consistently estimated by replacing $\boldsymbol{\psi} = (\lambda_1, \lambda_2)$ by $\boldsymbol{\psi} = (\hat{\lambda}_1, \hat{\lambda}_2)$. Let us denote the estimator by $\theta_{1,t_0}^{(CS)}(\tau; \hat{\boldsymbol{\psi}})$. By using the bivariate delta method, the variance of $\theta_{1,t_0}^{(CS)}(\tau; \hat{\boldsymbol{\psi}})$ can be directly evaluated from

$$\text{Var}\left[\theta_{1,t_0}^{(CS)}(\tau; \hat{\boldsymbol{\psi}})\right] = \left(\frac{\partial \theta_{1,t_0}^{(CS)}(\tau; \boldsymbol{\psi})}{\partial \boldsymbol{\psi}}\right)^T I_{(obs)}^{-1}(\boldsymbol{\psi}) \left(\frac{\partial \theta_{1,t_0}^{(CS)}(\tau; \boldsymbol{\psi})}{\partial \boldsymbol{\psi}}\right),$$

$$(4.20)$$

where

$$\left(\frac{\partial \theta_{1,t_0}^{(CS)}(\tau; \boldsymbol{\psi})}{\partial \boldsymbol{\psi}}\right)^T = \left(\frac{\partial \theta_{1,t_0}^{(CS)}(\tau; \boldsymbol{\psi})}{\partial \lambda_1}, \frac{\partial \theta_{1,t_0}^{(CS)}(\tau; \boldsymbol{\psi})}{\partial \lambda_2}\right)^T$$

$$= \left(\frac{1}{\lambda_1^2} \log\left(1 - \tau e^{-\lambda_2 t_0}\right), -\frac{\tau t_0 e^{-\lambda_2 t_0}}{\lambda_1(1 - \tau e^{-\lambda_2 t_0})}\right),$$

and $I_{(obs)}^{-1}(\boldsymbol{\psi})$ is a 2×2 variance–covariance matrix with diagonal elements of $\text{Var}(\hat{\lambda}_j) = \lambda_j^2 / \sum_{i=1}^n \delta_{ji}$ $(j = 1, 2)$ and off-diagonal elements of 0s. Therefore the variance of $\theta_{1,t_0}^{(CS)}(\tau; \hat{\boldsymbol{\psi}})$ simplifies to

$$\left(\frac{\lambda_1^2}{\sum_{i=1}^n \delta_{1i}}\right)\left\{\frac{1}{\lambda_1^2} \log\left(1 - \tau e^{-\lambda_2 t_0}\right)\right\}^2$$

$$+ \left(\frac{\lambda_2^2}{\sum_{i=1}^n \delta_{2i}}\right)\left\{\frac{\tau t_0 e^{-\lambda_2 t_0}}{\lambda_1(1 - \tau e^{-\lambda_2 t_0})}\right\}^2,$$

which can be again consistently estimated by replacing $\boldsymbol{\psi} = (\lambda_1, \lambda_2)$ by $\boldsymbol{\psi} = (\hat{\lambda}_1, \hat{\lambda}_2)$.

4.3.2 Independent Two-Sample Case

Suppose we are interested in comparing the quantiles from two residual life distributions under competing risks. Let us denote $\theta_{1,t_0}^{(k)}(\tau; \boldsymbol{\psi}^{(k)})$ for the τ-quantile from a residual life distribution of type 1 events for group k $(k = 1, 2)$ at time t_0. Because the estimator $\theta_{1,t_0}^{(k)}(\tau; \hat{\boldsymbol{\psi}}^{(k)})$ asymptotically follows the normal distribution with mean $\theta_{1,t_0}^{(k)}(\tau; \boldsymbol{\psi}^{(k)})$ and the variance given in (4.14) or in (4.20) for each group k, under the null hypothesis of H_0 : $\theta_{1,t_0}^{(1)}(\tau; \boldsymbol{\psi}^{(1)}) = \theta_{1,t_0}^{(2)}(\tau; \boldsymbol{\psi}^{(2)})$, a two-sample statistic can be constructed as

$$W_{1,t_0}(\tau) = \frac{\theta_{1,t_0}^{(1)}(\tau; \hat{\boldsymbol{\psi}}^{(1)}) - \theta_{1,t_0}^{(2)}(\tau; \hat{\boldsymbol{\psi}}^{(2)})}{\sqrt{\widehat{\text{Var}}\left[\theta_{1,t_0}(\tau; \hat{\boldsymbol{\psi}}^{(pooled)})\right] + \widehat{\text{Var}}\left[\theta_{1,t_0}(\tau; \hat{\boldsymbol{\psi}}^{(pooled)})\right]}},$$

$$(4.21)$$

where $\theta_{1,t_0}(\tau; \hat{\boldsymbol{\psi}}^{(pooled)})$ is the pooled estimate of the τ-quantile residual life for type 1 events. The test statistic (4.21) converges in distribution to the standard normal distribution with mean 0 and variance 1 by the Slutsky's theorem (Slutsky, 1925). Here note that $\widehat{\text{Var}}\left[\theta_{1,t_0}(\tau; \hat{\boldsymbol{\psi}}^{(pooled)})\right]$ is the consistent estimator for the variance of $\theta_{1,t_0}(\tau; \hat{\boldsymbol{\psi}}^{(pooled)})$. For a two-sided test, a small or large value of $W_{1,t_0}(\tau)$ would favor the rejection of the null hypothesis.

4.3.3   Parametric Regression

The parametric modeling under the popular proportional hazards model (Cox, 1972, 1975) often assumes the Weibull distribution as the baseline distribution, which is defined as the distribution with all the covariate values being 0. Under the competing risks, however, the baseline distribution could be improper. For example, consider a regression model with a single covariate coded 0 for placebo group and 1 for treatment group, and suppose that we are interested in comparing the distributions of time-to-breast-cancer-related deaths between the two groups. This implies that the baseline distribution of the time-to-breast-cancer-related deaths for the placebo group must be improper.

As presented for one-sample case in Sect. 4.3.1, in this section we will first consider inference on the regression coefficients and the baseline parameters. Then the delta method will be used to infer the τ-residual life quantile for type j events, which would be a function of those parameters.

Fine and Gray (1999) considered the proportional hazards model to directly infer the effects of covariates on the subdistribution hazard of type j events, which specifies that

$$\gamma_j(t; \boldsymbol{\beta}_j, \mathbf{z}) = \gamma_{j0}(t) \exp(\boldsymbol{\beta}'_j \mathbf{z}), \tag{4.22}$$

where the subdistribution hazard function was defined in (4.5), $\boldsymbol{\beta}_j$ is a $(p+1) \times 1$ parameter vector, and $\mathbf{z}$ is a time-independent $(p+1) \times 1$ covariate vector. Defining $g_j(v) = \log\{-\log(1-v)\}$, the model (4.22) can be expressed as the general transformation model

$$g_j\{F_j(t; \boldsymbol{\beta}_j, \mathbf{z})\} = u_j(t) + \boldsymbol{\beta}'_j \mathbf{z}, \quad j = 1, \ldots, J, \tag{4.23}$$

where $u_j(t) = \log\left\{\int_0^t \gamma_{j0}(v)dv\right\}$. Equivalently, the cumulative probability of a type j event is given by

$$F_j(t; \boldsymbol{\beta}_j, \mathbf{z}) = 1 - \exp\{-\exp(\boldsymbol{\beta}'_j \mathbf{z}) H_{j0}(t)\},$$

where $H_{j0}(t) = \int_0^t \gamma_{j0}(v)dv$ is the baseline cumulative hazard function for the subdistribution of type j events.

To allow for more flexibility, the link function $g_j(v)$ might take the odds rate transformation

$$g_j(v_j; \alpha_j) = \log[\{(1-v_j)^{-\alpha_j} - 1\}/\alpha_j], \quad -\infty < \alpha_j < \infty, \tag{4.24}$$

which includes the proportional hazards and proportional odds models (Dabrowska and Doksum, 1998) as special cases when $\alpha_j \to 0$ and $\alpha_j = 1$, respectively. Under model (4.23) with the link function (4.24), the cumulative probability of a type j event is given by

$$F_j(t; \alpha_j, \boldsymbol{\beta}_j, \mathbf{z}) = 1 - \{1 + \alpha_j \exp(\boldsymbol{\beta}'_j \mathbf{z}) H_{j0}(t)\}^{-1/\alpha_j}. \tag{4.25}$$

Jeong and Fine (2007) considered the two-parameter Gompertz distribution for the baseline distribution with the cumulative distribution function

$$F_{j0}^{(G2)}(t; \rho_j, \kappa_j) = 1 - \exp[\kappa_j\{1 - \exp(\rho_j t)\}/\rho_j], \tag{4.26}$$

where $-\infty < \rho_j < \infty$ and $0 < \kappa_j < \infty$. Note that an improper distribution occurs when $\rho_j < 0$ and $\kappa_j < \infty$. Under this distribution, the hazard function and the cumulative hazard function are given by $\gamma_{j0}^{(G2)}(t) = \kappa_j \exp(\rho_j t)$ and $H_{j0}^{(G2)}(t) = \kappa_j \{\exp(\rho_j t) - 1\}/\rho_j$, respectively.

It can be easily seen that the hazard function $\gamma_{j0}^{(G2)}(t)$ can fit only either increasing or decreasing hazards, but in practice the baseline hazard shape is often observed as unimodal or a U-shape. For example, Fig. 4.3 shows a plot of the estimated subdistribution hazard function from a breast cancer study when the events of interest is local or regional recurrence in the presence of other competing events such as distant recurrence, other types of cancer, or death prior to any disease.

To fit this type of unimodal subdistribution hazard shape, Haile (2008) extended the two-parameter Gompertz distribution to a three-parameter case. The three-parameter Gompertz distribution has the cumulative distribution function for type j events

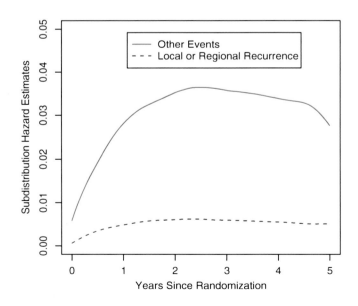

Fig. 4.3: Estimated unimodal subdistribution hazard shapes from a breast cancer study

$$F_{j0}^{(G3)}(t; \rho_j, \kappa_j, \eta_j) = 1 - \exp\left[-\left(\frac{\kappa_j}{\rho_j \eta_j}\right)\left\{\exp\left(\eta_j e^{\rho_j t}\right) - \exp(\eta_j)\right\}\right],$$
$$(4.27)$$

and hence the hazard function is

$$\gamma_{j0}^{(G3)}(t; \rho_j, \kappa_j, \eta_j) = \kappa_j \exp\{\rho_j t + \eta_j \exp(\rho_j t)\},$$

and the cumulative hazard function is

$$H_{j0}^{(G3)}(t; \rho_j, \kappa_j, \eta_j) = \left(\frac{\kappa_j}{\rho_j \eta_j}\right)\left\{\exp\left(\eta_j e^{\rho_j t}\right) - \exp(\eta_j)\right\}. \quad (4.28)$$

Figure 4.4 shows various shapes of the hazard function $\gamma_{j0}^{(G3)}$ $(t; \rho_j, \kappa_j, \eta_j)$ for different ρ_j values when κ_j and η_j are fixed as 1 and -0.25, respectively. The shapes include monotonely decreasing or increasing, and unimodal. In fact, the hazard function $\gamma_{j0}^{(G3)}(t; \rho_j, \kappa_j, \eta_j)$ reaches the maximum at $t = (1/\rho_j)\log(-1/\eta_j)$ implying its unimodality when $\eta_j < 0$.

As $t \to \infty$, the asymptote of $F_{j0}^{(G3)}(t; \rho_j, \kappa_j, \eta_j)$ approaches

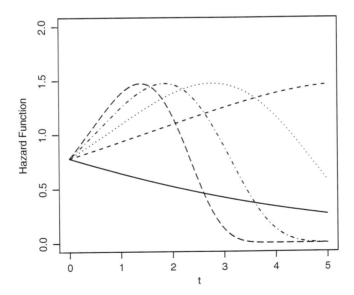

Fig. 4.4: Various hazard shapes from the three-parameter Gompertz distribution

$$\lim_{t\to\infty} F_{j0}^{(G3)}(t;\rho_j,\kappa_j,\eta_j) = 1 - \exp\left[\left(\frac{\kappa_j}{(\rho_j\eta_j)}\right)\{\exp(\eta_j) - 1\}\right], \rho_j < 0$$

$$= 1 - \exp\left\{\frac{\kappa_j \exp(\eta_j)}{(\rho_j\eta_j)}\right\}, \qquad \rho_j > 0, \eta_j < 0$$

$$= 1, \qquad\qquad \rho_j > 0, \eta_j > 0,$$

implying both proper and improper features in it.

Once it is determined which baseline distribution will be employed, the complete parametric form of $F_j(t;\mathbf{z})$ in (4.25) can also be determined. Suppose we have decided to adopt the three-parameter Gompertz distribution for the baseline. Then, by setting $\boldsymbol{\psi}_j = (\alpha_j, \boldsymbol{\beta}_j, \rho_j, \kappa_j, \eta_j)$, our parametric regression model will be given by

$$F_j(t;\boldsymbol{\psi}_j,\mathbf{z}) = 1 - \{1 + \alpha_j \exp(\boldsymbol{\beta}_j'\mathbf{z})H_{j0}^{(G3)}(t;\boldsymbol{\psi}_j)\}^{-1/\alpha_j}, \quad (4.29)$$

where $H_{j0}^{(G3)}(t;\boldsymbol{\psi}_j)$ was defined in (4.28).

We can now proceed with the usual maximum likelihood estimation under the parametric model (4.29). Let T_i and C_i be the potential failure time and the potential censoring time, respectively, for the ith subject. Define $X_i = \min(T_i, C_i)$. The indicator function for a type j event is

$$\delta_{ji} = 1, \text{ if the } i\text{th subject experiences a type } j \text{ event first}$$
$$0, \text{ otherwise,}$$

for $j = 1, \ldots, J$. For the simple case where there exist only two types of competing events as before, $\delta_{1i}=1$ if the ith subject experiences an event of interest as first event and 0 otherwise, and δ_{2i} is similarly defined for the ith subject experiencing competing events. Therefore the observable data can be denoted as $(X_i, \delta_{1i}, \delta_2, \mathbf{z}_i)$ $(i = 1, \ldots, n)$ in this case.

Following similar arguments for direct inference as in Sect. 4.3.1, given covariate $\mathbf{z}_i = \mathbf{z}_i$, the likelihood function in general is given by

$$\prod_{i=1}^{n}\left[\left\{\prod_{j=1}^{J}f_j(x_i;\boldsymbol{\psi}_j,\mathbf{z}_i)^{\delta_{ji}}\right\}\left\{1-\sum_{j=1}^{J}F_j(x_i;\boldsymbol{\psi}_j,\mathbf{z}_i)\right\}^{1-\sum_{j=1}^{J}\delta_{ji}}\right],$$

$$(4.30)$$

where $f_j(x;\boldsymbol{\psi}_j,\mathbf{z}_i)=dF_j(x;\boldsymbol{\psi}_j,\mathbf{z}_i)/dx$ $(j=1,\ldots,J)$. For the special case where there are only two types of competing events, the likelihood function (4.30) simplifies to

$$\prod_{i=1}^{n}f_1(x_i;\boldsymbol{\psi}_1,\mathbf{z}_i)^{\delta_{1i}}f_2(x_i;\boldsymbol{\psi}_2,\mathbf{z}_i)^{\delta_{2i}}\{1-F_1(x_i;\boldsymbol{\psi}_1,\mathbf{z}_i)-F_2(x_i;\boldsymbol{\psi}_2,\mathbf{z}_i)\}^{1-\delta_{1i}-\delta_{2i}}.$$

$$(4.31)$$

From (4.31), the log-likelihood function can be written as

$$\sum_{i=1}^{n}\left[\sum_{j=1}^{2}\delta_{ji}\log\{f_j(x_i,\boldsymbol{\psi}_j;\mathbf{z}_i)\}+\left(1-\sum_{j=1}^{2}\delta_{ji}\right)\log\left\{1-\sum_{j=1}^{2}F_j(x_i,\boldsymbol{\psi}_j;\mathbf{z}_i)\right\}\right].$$

$$(4.32)$$

Differentiating (4.32) and setting the resulting score function equal to 0 with respect to $\boldsymbol{\psi}=(\boldsymbol{\psi}_1^T,\boldsymbol{\psi}_2^T)^T$, the maximum likelihood estimator $\hat{\boldsymbol{\psi}}=(\hat{\boldsymbol{\psi}}_1,\hat{\boldsymbol{\psi}}_2)$ can be obtained. By the invariance property, the maximum likelihood estimator of $F_j(t;\boldsymbol{\psi}_j,\mathbf{z})$ is $F_j(t;\hat{\boldsymbol{\psi}}_j,\mathbf{z})$ $(j=1,2)$.

Now, by applying the formula (4.7) for the residual life cumulative incidence for type 1 events, given $\mathbf{z}_i=\mathbf{z}_i$, we have

$$F_{1,t_0}(t;\boldsymbol{\psi},\mathbf{z}_i)=\frac{F_1(t+t_0;\boldsymbol{\psi}_1,\mathbf{z}_i)-F_1(t_0;\boldsymbol{\psi}_1,\mathbf{z}_i)}{1-F_1(t_0;\boldsymbol{\psi}_1,\mathbf{z}_i)-F_2(t_0;\boldsymbol{\psi}_2,\mathbf{z}_i)},$$

which gives the τ-quantile function as

$$\theta_{1,t_0}(\tau;\boldsymbol{\psi},\mathbf{z}_i)=F_1^{-1}[F_1(t_0;\boldsymbol{\psi}_1,\mathbf{z}_i)+\tau\{1-F_1(t_0;\boldsymbol{\psi}_1,\mathbf{z}_i)-F_2(t_0;\boldsymbol{\psi}_2,\mathbf{z}_i)\};\boldsymbol{\psi}_1,\mathbf{z}_i]-t_0.$$

$$(4.33)$$

The τ-quantile residual life given covariates $\mathbf{z}_i$, $\theta_{1,t_0}(\tau;\boldsymbol{\psi},\mathbf{z}_i)$, can be estimated consistently by replacing $\boldsymbol{\psi}_j$ $(j=1,2)$ with their maximum likelihood estimates $\hat{\boldsymbol{\psi}}_j$ $(j=1,2)$ in (4.33), which will be denoted by $\theta_{1,t_0}(\tau; \hat{\psi}, \mathbf{z}_i)$. By the two-step delta method used in Sect. 4.3.1, the variance formula for $\theta_{1,t_0}(\tau; \hat{\psi}, \mathbf{z}_i)$ is given by

$$\text{Var}\left[\theta_{1,t_0}(\tau; \hat{\psi}, \mathbf{z}_i)\right] = \frac{\text{Var}\left[F_{1,t_0}(\theta_{1,t_0}(\tau; \psi, \mathbf{z}_i); \hat{\psi}, \mathbf{z}_i)\right]}{(f_{1,t_0}(\theta_{1,t_0}(\tau; \psi, \mathbf{z}_i); \psi, \mathbf{z}_i))^2}, \quad (4.34)$$

where

$$f_{1,t_0}(t; \psi, \mathbf{z}_i) = \frac{dF_{1,t_0}(t; \psi, \mathbf{z}_i)}{dt} = \frac{f_1(t + t_0; \psi_1, \mathbf{z}_i)}{1 - F_1(t_0; \psi_1, \mathbf{z}_i) - F_2(t_0; \psi_2, \mathbf{z}_i)},$$

and

$$\text{Var}\left[F_{1,t_0}(x; \hat{\psi}, \mathbf{z}_i)\right] = \left(\frac{\partial F_{1,t_0}(x; \psi, \mathbf{z}_i)}{\partial \psi}\right)' I_{(obs)}^{-1}(\psi) \left(\frac{\partial F_{1,t_0}(x; \psi, \mathbf{z}_i)}{\partial \psi}\right).$$

Here $\partial F_{1,t_0}(x; \psi, \mathbf{z}_i)/\partial \psi$ is a vector containing the first derivatives of the residual life cumulative incidence function $F_{1,t_0}(x; \psi, \mathbf{z}_i)$ with respect to the parameter vector ψ, and $I_{(obs)}^{-1}(\psi)$ is the observed information matrix for ψ, i.e. the negative second derivatives of the log-likelihood function (4.32) with respect to ψ. Given the covariate values $\mathbf{z}_i$, the variance formula (4.34) can be consistently estimated by replacing ψ, $\theta_{1,t_0}(\tau; \psi, \mathbf{z}_i)$, and $f_{1,t_0}(\theta_{1,t_0}(\tau; \psi, \mathbf{z}_i); \psi, \mathbf{z}_i)$ with the maximum likelihood estimates $\hat{\psi}$, $\theta_{1,t_0}(\tau; \hat{\psi}, \mathbf{z}_i)$, and $f_{1,t_0}(\theta_{1,t_0}(\tau; \hat{\psi}, \mathbf{z}_i); \hat{\psi}, \mathbf{z}_i)$.

4.4 Nonparametric Inference

The parametric inference procedures considered in the previous sections would be useful and more accurate when an assumed parametric distribution fits the data well. However, the more flexible the adopted distribution is, the more parameters to be estimated, especially under a regression model with competing risks, which would make the surface of the likelihood function flatter, and hence difficult to find the global maximum. The nonparametric procedures can often overcome this hurdle at the cost of minimal efficiency loss. In this section, we review the nonparametric and semiparametric methods recently developed for inference on the quantile residual life function.

4.4.1 One-Sample Case

Under competing risks, the cause-specific τ-quantile residual lifetime can be inferred once the residual life subdistribution of type j events of interest is specified. The subdistribution function of type j residual lifetimes at time t_0 was defined as (Jeong and Fine, 2009)

$$
\begin{aligned}
F_{j,t_0}(t) &\equiv \Pr(T - t_0 \le t, \epsilon = j | T > t_0) \\
&= \{F_j(t + t_0) - F_j(t_0)\}/S(t_0), \quad t > t_0, \quad (4.35)
\end{aligned}
$$

where $F_j(t) = \Pr(T \le t, \epsilon = j)$ is the cause j cumulative incidence function and $S(\cdot)$ is the all-cause survival function. The residual cumulative incidence function $F_{j,t_0}(t)$ can be nonparametrically estimated by replacing $F_j(\cdot)$ by the estimate given in (4.4) and $S(\cdot)$ by the Kaplan–Meier estimates.

Again for simplicity, it will be assumed that there are only two types of competing events other than independently censored observations, denoted as type 1 and type 2, where the type 1 events are of primary interest. Then the estimating equation for the τ-quantile residual lifetime for the subdistribution of type 1 events, $\theta_{1,t_0}(\tau)$, can be expressed as

$$
u(\theta_{1,t_0}(\tau)) = \hat{F}_1(t_0 + \theta_{1,t_0}(\tau)) - \hat{F}_1(t_0) - \tau \hat{S}(t_0) = 0, \quad (4.36)
$$

where $\hat{F}_1(\cdot)$ is an empirical estimate of the cumulative incidence function for type 1 events, $F_1(\cdot)$, and $\hat{S}(\cdot)$ is the Kaplan–Meier estimates for the all-cause survival function, $S(\cdot)$. Solving Eq. (4.36) provides the estimate of $\theta_{1,t_0}(\tau)$ as

$$
\hat{\theta}_{1,t_0}(\tau) = \hat{F}_1^{-1}\left(\hat{F}_1(t_0) + \tau \hat{S}(t_0)\right) - t_0. \quad (4.37)
$$

Jeong and Fine (2009) showed that the estimate $\hat{\theta}_{1,t_0}(\tau)$ is uniformly consistent for all τ such that $\theta_{1,t0}(\tau) < \infty$ and $n^{1/2}[\hat{\theta}_{1,t_0}(\tau) - \theta_{1,t_0}(\tau)]$ converges weakly to a Gaussian process whose variance depends on improper probability density function for cause-specific events. To avoid the difficulty in estimating the improper probability density function nonparametrically, Jeong and Fine (2009) proposed to use an inference procedure based on the estimating equation (4.36) itself.

Let us first define some notations under the competing risks martingale framework. Let T_i $(i = 1, \ldots, n)$ be failure times with survivor function $S(t)$ and cumulative hazard function $\Lambda(t) = -\log S(t)$. Because of early termination of study, or loss to follow-up, T_i may not be completely observed. In conjunction with the event time T_i, let C_i be the censoring time. Then, for a subject i, we observe $\{(X_i, \delta_i), i = 1, \ldots, n\}$, where $\delta_i = \epsilon_i I(T_i \leq C_i)$ and $X_i = \min(T_i, C_i)$. Recall that $\epsilon_i = 1, 2$ is an index for the event type for the ith subject.

Suppose that $Y_i(t)=I(X_i \geq t)$ and $N_i(t)=I(T_i \leq C_i)I(X_i \leq t)$ are the individual at-risk and event processes associated with all causes, respectively. For the cause-specific events of type 1, we define the event process as $N_1^i(t) = I(T_i \leq C_i, \delta_i = 1)I(X_i \leq t)$. Also define $y(t) = \lim_{n \to \infty} \sum_{i=1}^{n} Y_i(t)/n$ to be the limiting at-risk process, and $M_1^i(t) = N_1^i(t) - \int_0^t Y_i(v)d\Lambda_1(v)$, $\Lambda_1(v)$ being the cause-specific cumulative hazard function for type 1 events, and $M_i(t) = N_i(t) - \int_0^t Y_i(v)d\Lambda(v)$ to be the cause-specific and all-cause martingale processes, respectively. The total all-cause and cause 1 counting processes are denoted as $N(t) = \sum_{i=1}^{n} N_i(t)$ and $N_1(t) = \sum_{i=1}^{n} N_1^i(t)$, respectively.

Using the martingale representations of the cumulative incidence function (Aalen, 1978; Andersen *et al.*, 1993; Pepe, 1991) and survival function (Andersen *et al.*, 1993), Jeong and Fine (2013) showed that $u(\theta_{1,t_0}(\tau))$ follows an asymptotically normal distribution with mean 0 and variance $\sum_{i=1}^{n} \zeta_i^2$, where

$$\zeta_i = \int_{t_0}^{t_0+\theta_{1,t_0}(\tau)} \frac{S(v)}{ny(v)} dM_1^i(v) - \int_{t_0}^{t_0+\theta_{1,t_0}(\tau)} S(v) \left\{ \int_0^v \frac{dM_1^i(s)}{ny(s)} \right\} dv$$
$$- \tau S(t_0) \int_0^{t_0} \frac{dM_i(s)}{ny(s)},$$

which can be consistently estimated by

$$
\begin{aligned}
\hat{\zeta}_i &= \int_{t_0}^{t_0+\hat{\theta}_{1,t_0}(\tau)} \frac{\hat{S}(v)}{Y(v)} d\hat{M}_1^i(v) - \int_{t_0}^{t_0+\hat{\theta}_{1,t_0}(\tau)} \hat{S}(v) \left\{ \int_0^v \frac{d\hat{M}_1^i(s)}{Y(s)} \right\} dv \\
&\quad -\tau \hat{S}(t_0) \int_0^{t_0} \frac{d\hat{M}_i(s)}{Y(s)},
\end{aligned} \tag{4.38}
$$

where

$$
\hat{M}_1^i(t) = N_1^i(t) - \int_0^t Y_i(v) d\hat{\Lambda}_1(v), \qquad \hat{\Lambda}_1(v) = \int_0^v \frac{dN_1(s)}{Y(s)}
$$

and

$$
\hat{M}_i(t) = N_i(t) - \int_0^t Y_i(v) d\hat{\Lambda}(v), \qquad \hat{\Lambda}(v) = \int_0^v \frac{dN(s)}{Y(s)}.
$$

We will denote $\widehat{\mathrm{Var}}\left[u\left(\hat{\theta}_{1,t_0}(\tau)\right)\right] = \sum_{i=1}^n \hat{\zeta}_i^2$ for the consistent estimate of the variance of $u\left(\theta_{1,t_0}(\tau)\right)$. Therefore, the test statistic

$$
u^2\left(\hat{\theta}_{1,t_0}(\tau)\right) / \widehat{\mathrm{Var}}\left[u\left(\hat{\theta}_{1,t_0}(\tau)\right)\right]
$$

follows a χ^2-distribution with 1 degree of freedom, which can be inverted to obtain the $100\times(1-\alpha)\%$ confidence interval for $\theta_{1,t_0}(\tau)$, i.e.

$$
\{\theta_{1,t_0}(\tau) : u^2\left(\theta_{1,t_0}(\tau)\right) / \widehat{\mathrm{Var}}\left[u\left(\hat{\theta}_{1,t_0}(\tau)\right)\right] < \chi^2_{1-\alpha,1}\}, \tag{4.39}
$$

where $\chi^2_{1-\alpha,1}$ is the $(1-\alpha)$-percentile of the χ^2-distribution with 1 degree of freedom.

Example 4.3. For the illustrative purpose, we have simulated a dataset following the same steps from Jeong and Fine (2013). Specifically, we have used the following model to generate the dataset:

$$
\begin{aligned}
F_j(t) &= \Pr(T \le t, \epsilon = j) \\
&= \Pr(\epsilon = j)\Pr(T \le t | \epsilon = j) \\
&= \pi_j \left\{1 - \exp(-\lambda_j t^{\kappa_j})\right\}, \tag{4.40}
\end{aligned}
$$

where π_j is a leveling-off parameter for the type j subdistribution, so that $\pi_1 + \pi_2 = 1$ without censoring, and λ_j and κ_j are scale and index parameters for the assumed Weibull distribution, respectively. Therefore first one can simulate the event type indicator ϵ (=1 or 2) from a Bernoulli distribution with success probability of π_j, and then conditional on the ϵ value, an event time is generated from the proper Weibull distribution $F_j(t)/\pi_j$. The independent censoring variable C is assumed to follow a uniform distribution between 0 and c, where the constant c controls the censoring proportion.

The simulated dataset of size 10 consists of observed event or follow-up time x_i=(0.504, 0.974, 1.326, 1.358, 2.309, 2.577, 3.425, 3.666, 5.524, 11.482) and the event type indicator δ_i=(2, 1, 0, 1, 2, 1, 2, 1, 2, 2), where 1=type 1, 2=type 2, and 0=censored.

Figure 4.5 shows the cumulative incidence estimates for each event type. For ordered survival times, $x_{(i)}$ ($i = 1, 2, \ldots, 10$), Table 4.1 shows the estimated cumulative incidence functions for type 1 events ($\hat{F}_1(x_{(i)})$) and type 2 events ($\hat{F}_2(x_{(i)})$), and the Kaplan–Meier estimates ($\hat{S}(x_{(i)})$) based on both types of events.

Now suppose that we are interested in estimating the 0.2-quantile residual lifetime of the subdistribution of type 1 events at $t_0 = 2$. From Table 4.1 and Fig. 4.5, since $\hat{F}_1(2) = 0.214$ and $\hat{S}(2) = 0.686$, Eq. (4.37) gives

$$
\begin{aligned}
\hat{\theta}_{1,2}(0.2) &= \hat{F}_1^{-1}\left(\hat{F}_1(2) + 0.2 \times \hat{S}(2)\right) - 2 \\
&= \hat{F}_1^{-1}\left(0.214 + 0.2 \times 0.686\right) - 2 \\
&= \hat{F}_1^{-1}\left(0.351\right) - 2 = 3.666 - 2 = 1.666.
\end{aligned}
$$

To estimate the variance of $u(\hat{\theta}_{1,2}(0.2))$, we need to re-express (4.38) in a discrete version. Noting that the jump size of the counting process of type 1 event for the subject i, $dN_1^i(t)$, equals 1 at $t = x_{(i)}$ only with $\delta_{(i)} = 1$, Eq. (4.38) can be rewritten as

$$
\begin{aligned}
\hat{\zeta}_i &= I_{[t_0, t_0 + \hat{q}]}(t_{(i)}) \frac{\hat{S}(t_{(i)}) dN_1^i(t_{(i)})}{Y(t_{(i)})} \\
&\quad - \sum_{j=1}^{n} I_{[t_0, t_0 + \hat{q}]}(t_{(j)}) \frac{\hat{S}(t_{(j)}) dN_1(t_{(j)})}{Y(t_{(j)})^2}
\end{aligned}
$$

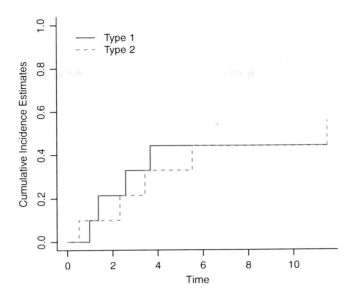

Fig. 4.5: The cumulative incidence estimates from the simulated dataset

$$-(t_{(i)} - t_{(i-1)})\hat{S}(t_{(i-1)}) \left\{ \frac{I_{[t_0,t_0+\hat{q}]}(t_{(i)})dN_1^i(t_{(i)})}{Y(t_{(i)})} \right.$$

$$\left. - \sum_{j=1}^n I_{[t_0,t_0+\hat{q}]}(t_{(j)}) \frac{dN_1(t_{(j)})}{Y(t_{(j)})^2} \right\}$$

$$-\tau\hat{S}(t_0) \left\{ \frac{I_{[0,t_0]}(t_{(i)})dN_i(t_{(i)})}{Y(t_{(i)})} - \sum_{j=1}^n I_{[0,t_0]}(t_{(j)}) \frac{dN(t_{(j)})}{Y(t_{(j)})^2} \right\},$$

where $\hat{q} = \hat{\theta}_{1,2}(0.2)$. Recall that in our numerical example above, $\hat{q} = 1.666$. Table 4.2 completes all the components required to calculate the variance estimate.

Therefore the first term of $\hat{\zeta}_i$ can be calculated from

$$\hat{\zeta}_{i,1} = \frac{\hat{S}(t_{(i)})dN_1^i(t_{(i)})}{Y(t_{(i)})} - \sum_{j=5}^{\min(i,3.666)} \left(\frac{\hat{S}(x_{(j)})dN_1(x_{(j)})}{Y(x_{(j)})^2} \right),$$

which generates a vector of 0.0, 0.073, -0.018, 0.033, -0.044, and -0.044 for $i = 5,\ldots, 10$, respectively. Similarly the second term can be calculated from

Table 4.1: A simulated dataset under competing risks: $x_{(i)}$, ordered survival times; $\delta_{(i)}=1$ for type 1 events, 2 for type 2 events, and 0 for censored; $\widehat{F}_1(x_{(i)})$, the cumulative incidence estimates for type 1 events; $\widehat{F}_2(x_{(i)})$, the cumulative incidence estimates for type 2 events; $\widehat{S}(x_{(i)})$, the Kaplan–Meier estimates based on both types of events

i	$x_{(i)}$	$\delta_{(i)}$	$\widehat{F}_1(t_{(i)})$	$\widehat{F}_2(t_{(i)})$	$\widehat{S}(t_{(i)})$
1	0.504	2	0.000	0.100	0.900
2	0.974	1	0.100	0.100	0.800
3	1.326	0	0.100	0.100	0.800
4	1.358	1	0.214	0.100	0.686
5	2.309	2	0.214	0.214	0.571
6	2.577	1	0.329	0.214	0.457
7	3.425	2	0.329	0.329	0.343
8	3.666	1	0.443	0.329	0.229
9	5.524	2	0.443	0.443	0.114
10	11.482	2	0.443	0.557	0.000

$$\hat{\zeta}_{i,2} = (x_{(i)}-x_{(i-1)})\hat{S}(x_{(i-1)})\left\{\frac{dN_1^i(x_{(i)})}{Y(x_{(i)})} - \sum_{j=5}^{\min(i,3.666)}\left(\frac{dN_1(x_{(j)})}{Y(x_{(j)})^2}\right)\right\},$$

which gives a vector of 0.0, 0.025, -0.016, 0.015, -0.064, and -0.103 for $i = 5,\ldots,$ 10, respectively. Lastly, the third term simplifies to

$$\hat{\zeta}_{i,3} = 0.2\hat{S}(2)\left\{\frac{dN_i(t_{(i)})}{Y(t_{(i)})} - \sum_{j=5}^{\min(i,2)}\left(\frac{dN(t_{(j)})}{Y(t_{(j)})^2}\right)\right\},$$

which gives 0.012, 0.012, -0.003, 0.014, -0.006, -0.006, -0.006, -0.006, -0.006, and -0.006, for $i = 1, .., 10$. Finally the variance of $u(\hat{\theta}_{1,2}(0.2))$ can be calculated as

$$\text{Var}[u(\hat{\theta}_{1,2}(0.2))] = \sum_{i=1}^{10}\hat{\zeta}_i^2 = \sum_{i=1}^{10}(\hat{\zeta}_{i,1} - \hat{\zeta}_{i,2} - \hat{\zeta}_{i,3})^2 = 0.0090.$$

Table 4.2: Quantities required for variance calculation; $I_1 = I_{[t_0,t_0+\hat{q}]}(x_{(i)})$, $I_2 = I_{[0,t_0]}(x_{(i)})$

(i)	$Y(x_{(i)})$	I_1	I_2	$dN(x_{(i)})$	$dN_1(x_{(i)})$	$x_{(i)} - x_{(i-1)}$	$\hat{S}(x_{(i-1)})$
1	10	0	1	1	0	0.504	1.000
2	9	0	1	1	1	0.470	0.900
3	8	0	1	0	0	0.352	0.800
4	7	0	1	1	1	0.384	0.800
5	6	1	0	1	0	0.951	0.686
6	5	1	0	1	1	0.268	0.571
7	4	1	0	1	0	0.848	0.457
8	3	1	0	1	1	0.241	0.343
9	2	0	0	1	0	1.858	0.229
10	1	0	0	1	0	5.958	0.114

The 95% confidence interval can be obtained by inverting (4.39) as a function of $q = \theta_{1,2}(0.2)$, which gave a noninformative 95% confidence interval $(-\infty, \infty)$ in this case due to the small sample size. To see a better picture, the sample size was increased to 100. Figure 4.6 shows the numerical evaluation of one-sample statistic for the 0.2-quantile of the residual life distribution of type 1 events at time $t_0 = 2$. The estimated 0.2-quantile in this case was 2.361 and associated 95% confidence interval was $(0.87, 4.21)$ by inverting the curve in Fig. 4.6 at the dashed line, which is the 95th percentile of a χ^2-distribution with 1 degree of freedom.

R codes used to generate the dataset and to perform data analysis presented in this example are provided in Appendix A.4.

4.4.2 Independent Two-Sample Case

The results established for one-sample case in the previous section can be extended directly to the two-sample case. Suppose that n_k patients are randomized to group k $(k = 1, 2)$, so that the total number of patients is $n = n_1 + n_2$, and we want to compare

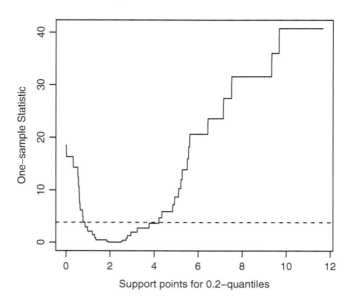

Fig. 4.6: Estimation of 95% confidence interval for the true 0.2-quantile for the residual life distribution of type 1 events by inverting one-sample test statistic when sample size is 100

the τ-residual lifetimes from subdistributions of type 1 events between two groups at time t_0. For group k, let $\theta_{1,t_0}^{(k)}(\tau)$ be the true τ-percentile residual lifetime of the subdistribution of type 1 events at time t_0. Suppose we are interested in making inference through the ratio of two τ-percentile residual lifetimes, i.e. $r_{1,t_0} = \theta_{1,t_0}^{(2)}(\tau)/\theta_{1,t_0}^{(1)}(\tau)$. A statistical hypothesis can be formulated as $H_0 : r_{1,t_0} = r_{1,t_0}^{(0)}$ vs. $H_1 : r_{1,t_0} \neq r_{1,t_0}^{(0)}$, where $r_{1,t_0}^{(0)}$ is a specified value of r_{1,t_0} associated with type 1 events under the null hypothesis. When $r_{1,t_0}^{(0)} = 1$, the equality of the two τ-quantile residual lifetimes at a given time t_0 will be tested. For group k, let the estimating function be

$$\hat{u}_k(\theta_{1,t_0}^{(k)}(\tau)) = \hat{F}_1^{(k)}\left(t_0 + \theta_{1,t_0}^{(k)}(\tau)\right) - \hat{F}_1^{(k)}(t_0) - p\hat{S}^{(k)}(t_0).$$

Noticing that $\theta_{1,t_0}^{(2)}(\tau) = r_{1,t_0}^{(0)}\theta_{1,t_0}^{(1)}(\tau)$ under $H_0 : r_{1,t_0} = r_{1,t_0}^{(0)}$, Jeong and Fine (2013) considered a two-sample test statistic for r_{1,t_0} as

$$V_{1,t_0}\left(r_{1,t_0}^{(0)}, \theta_{1,t_0}^{(1)}(\tau)\right) = \frac{\hat{u}_1^2\left(\theta_{1,t_0}^{(1)}(\tau)\right)}{\sum_{i=1}^n\left\{\hat{\zeta}_i^{(1)}\right\}^2} + \frac{\hat{u}_2^2\left(r_{1,t_0}^{(0)}\theta_{1,t_0}^{(1)}(\tau)\right)}{\sum_{i=1}^n\left\{\hat{\zeta}_i^{(2)}\right\}^2}, \quad (4.41)$$

where $\hat{\zeta}_i^{(k)}$ $(k = 1, 2)$ is similarly defined as in (4.38) for group k.

The statistic (4.41) would be still a function of the nuisance parameter $\theta_{1,t_0}^{(1)}(\tau)$, even though $r_{1,t_0}^{(0)}$ will be known under the null hypothesis. One way of eliminating the nuisance parameter would be to minimize the statistic over it. Following similar arguments as in Jeong $et\ al.$ (2007, Web Appendix), for any given time t_0 it can be shown that

$$W_{1,t_0}(r_{1,t_0}^{(0)}) = \inf_{\theta_{1,t_0}^{(1)}(\tau)} V_{1,t_0}\left(r_{1,t_0}^{(0)}, \theta_{1,t_0}^{(1)}(\tau)\right) \quad (4.42)$$

follows asymptotically a χ^2-distribution with 1 degree of freedom. We reject the null hypothesis $H_0 : r_{1,t_0} = r_{1,t_0}^{(0)}$ with type I error probability of α if $W_{1,t_0}(r_{1,t_0}^{(0)}) > \chi_{1,1-\alpha}^2$. Recall that an important advantage of using this type of statistic is that there is no need for estimating the underlying probability density function of a cause-specific failure time subdistribution under competing risks to make inference about the ratio of the two median residual lifetimes.

A $100\times(1 - \alpha)\%$ confidence interval for r_{1,t_0} can be obtained from

$$\{r_{1,t_0} : \inf_{\theta_{1,t_0}^{(1)}(\tau)} V_{1,t_0}\left(r_{1,t_0}, \theta_{1,t_0}^{(1)}(\tau)\right) < \chi_{1,1-\alpha}^2\}. \quad (4.43)$$

Note that, to achieve a confidence interval from (4.43), the statistic $V_{1,t_0}\left(r_{1,t_0}, \theta_{1,t_0}^{(1)}(\tau)\right)$ needs to be minimized over $\theta_{1,t_0}^{(1)}(\tau)$ for each fixed value of r_{1,t_0}. Thus values of r_{1,t_0} associated with the minimum values of the statistic that exceeds the value of $\chi_{1,1-\alpha}^2$ will be the lower and upper limits of the confidence interval.

To accommodate variability of the quantile residual lifetimes in the population by such as age at diagnosis of breast cancer, a stratified test statistic can also be constructed. Denoting L to be the number of strata, the stratified test statistic can be formed as

$$A_{1,t_0}(r_{1,t_0}^{(0)}) = \sum_{l=1}^L W_{1,t_0}^{(l)}(r_{1,t_0}^{(0)}),$$

where $W_{1,t_0}^{(l)}(r_{1,t_0}^{(0)})$ is the statistic $W_{1,t_0}(r_{1,t_0}^{(0)})$ that corresponds to the lth stratum. The statistic $A_{1,t_0}(r_{1,t_0}^{(0)})$ will asymptotically follow a χ^2-distribution with L degrees of freedom.

Example 4.4 (Confidence Interval for the Quantile Ratio). We have generated two datasets for groups 1 and 2 from the same distribution used for one-sample case with a sample size of 100 for each group. Suppose we are interested in testing the null hypothesis of $H_0 : r_{1,2} = 1$, where $r_{1,2} = \theta_{1,2}^{(2)}(0.2)/\theta_{1,2}^{(1)}(0.2)$ is the ratio of two 0.2-quantile residual lifetimes for the distribution of type 1 events at a given time $t_0 = 2$. The estimated 0.2-quantile residual lifetimes from the simulated dataset were $\hat{\theta}_{1,2}^{(1)}(0.2) = 2.36$ for group 1 and $\hat{\theta}_{1,2}^{(2)}(0.2) = 2.34$ for group 2, respectively, so that the estimated ratio was 0.99, close to 1 as expected. The variances of $u(\hat{\theta}_{1,2}^{(1)}(0.2))$ and $u(\hat{\theta}_{1,2}^{(2)}(0.2))$ can be calculated similarly as in Example 4.3. The test statistic (4.42) gives the value of $0.021 < \chi_{0.95,1}^2 = 3.841$, where $\chi_{0.95,1}^2$ is the 95th percentile of a χ^2-distribution with 1 degree of freedom, suggesting a lack of statistical evidence to reject the null hypothesis. Figure 4.7 shows the numerical evaluation of the statistic given in (4.43) as a function of $r_{1,2}$. A 95% confidence interval for $r_{1,2}$ can be obtained as (0.44, 2.93) by inverting the curve in Fig. 4.7 at the dashed line.

R codes used to generate the dataset and to perform data analysis presented in this example are provided in Appendix A.5.

Example 4.5 (Application to NSABP B-04 Dataset). Jeong and Fine (2009, 2013) applied the nonparametric methods of one-sample and two-sample inference on the quantile residual lifetimes under competing risks developed in Sects. 4.4.1 and 4.4.2 to the NSABP B-04 dataset. Competing events were deaths following breast cancer recurrence (both ipsilateral and contralateral) vs. non-breast-cancer-related deaths. They estimated 0.1-, 0.2-, and 0.3-quantile residual lifetimes to breast-cancer-related deaths and non-breast-cancer-related deaths in node-negative and node-positive patients, and then the ratio of the quantiles of the cause-specific residual life distributions was compared between the two

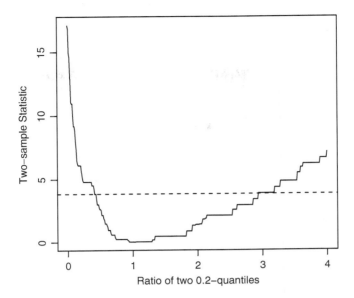

Fig. 4.7: Estimation of 95% confidence interval for the true ratio (=1) of two 0.2-quantiles for the residual life distributions of type 1 events by inverting two-sample test statistic when sample size is 100 per group

nodal groups. Table 4.3, extracted from Jeong and Fine (2013), summarizes the estimated τ-quantile residual lifetimes of *breast-cancer-related-deaths* in node-negative and node-positive groups, their ratios, and 95% confidence intervals for the ratios. As shown in Table 4.3, statistical analysis based on the quantiles provides more specific information about a distribution being inferred. For example, 4 years after surgery, the 0.3-quantile of the residual lifetime distribution of breast-cancer-related deaths in node-negative and node-positive populations was estimated as about 16 and 6 years, respectively, with the ratio of 0.35 (95% CI; 0.26–0.53) indicating a significant difference. The magnitudes of differences between the two quantile residual lifetimes vary for different time points and quantiles. The choice of a specific quantile to be reported may depend on the investigator's scientific and clinical interests. For example, an investigator may be interested in comparing two cause-specific quantile residual lifetimes among pa-

Table 4.3:   Estimated τ-percentile residual lifetimes of *breast-cancer-related-deaths* in node-negative and node-positive groups, the ratios, and 95% confidence intervals for the ratios (Jeong and Fine, 2013, *Biometrical Journal*)

t_0	τ	Quantile residual lifetime Node-negative	Node-positive	Ratio	95% CI
0	0.1	2.72	1.28	0.47	(0.42, 0.57)
	0.2	5.26	2.36	0.45	(0.37, 0.56)
	0.3	10.53	4.07	0.39	(0.29, 0.50)
2	0.1	1.95	1.04	0.53	(0.37, 0.74)
	0.2	4.81	2.76	0.57	(0.41, 0.75)
	0.3	11.45	4.98	0.43	(0.34, 0.54)
4	0.1	2.63	1.73	0.66	(0.40, 1.12)
	0.2	7.87	3.16	0.40	(0.31, 0.57)
	0.3	16.03	5.63	0.35	(0.26, 0.53)
6	0.1	3.96	1.04	0.26	(0.15, 0.41)
	0.2	9.99	2.98	0.30	(0.19, 0.45)
	0.3	21.41	6.77	0.32	(0.17, 0.55)
8	0.1	4.92	2.17	0.44	(0.24, 0.71)
	0.2	11.8	6.57	0.56	(0.30, 0.91)
	0.3	–	–	–	–

tients least affected by a study drug, e.g. using the 0.1-quantile of a subdistribution of time to events of interest while another investigator might be interested in comparing patients with better prognosis by using higher percentiles.

4.4.3   Semiparametric Regression

It would be useful to have a regression model that associates a set of covariates with the τ-quantile of a residual life distribution at time t_0 of a cause-specific event of interest in the presence of other competing events. For example, investigators might be interested in knowing a treatment effect on the median residual lifetime of the distribution of breast-cancer-related deaths in the presence of non-breast-cancer-related deaths such as cardiac deaths, adjusting for age and tumor size. We have considered a τ-quantile residual life regression model in Sect. 3.6, which will be extended here to the competing risks setting.

Without loss of generality, it will be assumed that there are only two types of events, i.e. type 1 and type 2, as before. Also let X_i, $i = 1, 2, \ldots, n$, denote the minimum of the failure time T_i and censoring time C_i, and let ϵ_i indicate the cause of failure and $\delta_i = I(T_i \leq C_i)\epsilon_i$.

Without censoring, for subject i, we define the conditional cumulative incidence function for the residual life distribution of type 1 events at time t_0, given a vector of covariates $\mathbf{z}_i$, as

$$
\begin{aligned}
F_{1,t_0}(t|\mathbf{z}_i) &\equiv \Pr(T_i - t_0 \leq t, \epsilon = 1 | T_i > t_0, \mathbf{z}_i) \\
&= \{F_1(t + t_0|\mathbf{z}_i) - F_1(t_0|\mathbf{z}_i)\}/S(t_0|\mathbf{z}_i), \quad t > t_0.
\end{aligned}
$$

Setting this equal to τ gives the equation for the τ-quantile residual lifetime for type 1 events, $\theta_{1,t_0}(\tau|\mathbf{z}_i)$, given the covariates $\mathbf{z}_i$, as

$$
u_0(\theta_{1,t_0}(\tau|\mathbf{z}_i)) = F_1(t_0 + \theta_{1,t_0}(\tau|\mathbf{z}_i)|\mathbf{z}_i) - F_1(t_0|\mathbf{z}_i) - \tau S(t_0|\mathbf{z}_i) = 0.
\tag{4.44}
$$

Similarly as in Sect. 3.6, $\theta_{1,t_0}(\tau|\mathbf{z}_i)$ in (4.44) can be formulated as log-linear in $\mathbf{z}_i$, i.e.

$$
\theta_{1,t_0}(\tau|\mathbf{z}_i) = \exp(\boldsymbol{\beta}'_{1,\tau|t_0}\mathbf{z}_i),
$$

where formally $\boldsymbol{\beta}_{1,\tau|t_0}$ is a $(p + 1) \times 1$ vector of the regression coefficients, and $\mathbf{z}_i$ is a $(p + 1) \times 1$ vector of covariates. Then Eq. (4.44) implies

$$
\begin{aligned}
&\Pr(T_i \leq t_0 + \exp(\boldsymbol{\beta}'_{1,\tau|t_0}\mathbf{z}_i), \epsilon_i = 1|\mathbf{z}_i) - \Pr(T_i \leq t_0, \epsilon_i = 1|\mathbf{z}_i) \\
&= \tau \Pr(T_i > t_0|\mathbf{z}_i).
\end{aligned}
\tag{4.45}
$$

Assuming conditional independence between (T_i, ϵ_i) and C_i given $\mathbf{z}_i$ (Peng and Fine, 2007), the first term of the left-hand side of Eq. (4.45) has the following equivalence:

$$E\left\{\frac{I(X_i \le t_0 + \exp(\boldsymbol{\beta}'_{1,\tau|t_0}\mathbf{z}_i), \delta_i = 1)}{G(X_i - |\mathbf{z}_i)}\Big|\mathbf{z}_i\right\}$$

$$= E\left[E\left\{\frac{I(T_i \le t_0 + \exp(\boldsymbol{\beta}'_{1,\tau|t_0}\mathbf{z}_i), \epsilon_i = 1, C_i \ge T_i)}{G(T_i - |\mathbf{z}_i)}\Big|T_i, \epsilon_i, \mathbf{z}_i\right\}\Big|\mathbf{z}_i\right]$$

$$= E\left[\frac{I(T_i \le t_0 + \exp(\boldsymbol{\beta}'_{1,\tau|t_0}\mathbf{z}_i), \epsilon = 1)G(T_i - |\mathbf{z}_i)}{G(T_i - |\mathbf{z}_i)}\Big|\mathbf{z}_i\right]$$

$$= \Pr(T_i \le t_0 + \exp(\boldsymbol{\beta}'_{1,\tau|t_0}\mathbf{z}_i), \epsilon_i = 1|\mathbf{z}_i),$$

where $G(t-)$ is the survival function of the censoring distribution just prior to t. Similarly, the second term of the left-hand side in Eq. (4.45) satisfies

$$\Pr(T_i \le t_0, \epsilon_i = 1|\mathbf{z}_i) = E\left\{\frac{I(X_i \le t_0, \delta_i = 1)}{G(X_i - |\mathbf{z}_i)}\Big|\mathbf{z}_i\right\}.$$

Therefore Eq. (4.45) can be re-expressed as

$$E\left[\frac{\left[I\{X_i \le t_0 + \exp(\boldsymbol{\beta}'_{1,\tau|t_0}\mathbf{z}_i)\} - I(X_i \le t_0)\right]I(\delta_i = 1)}{G(X_i - |\mathbf{z}_i)}\Big|\mathbf{z}_i\right]$$

$$= E\left\{\tau\frac{I(X_i > t_0)}{G(t_0|\mathbf{z}_i)}\Big|\mathbf{z}_i\right\},$$

which, following similar arguments as in Sect. 3.6.3, leads to an estimating equation for the regression parameter $\boldsymbol{\beta}_{1,\tau|t_0}$ (Lim, 2011),

$$\mathbf{S}_{1,t_0|\tau,n}(\boldsymbol{\beta}_{1,\tau|t_0}) = 0, \tag{4.46}$$

where $\mathbf{S}_{1,t_0|\tau,n}(\boldsymbol{\beta}_{1,\tau|t_0})$ is defined as

$$\sum_{i=1}^{n}\mathbf{z}_i\left[\frac{\left[I\{X_i \le t_0 + \exp(\boldsymbol{\beta}'_{1,\tau|t_0}\mathbf{z}_i)\} - I(X_i \le t_0)\right]I(\delta_i = 1)}{\hat{G}(X_i - |\mathbf{z}_i)} - \tau\frac{I(X_i > t_0)}{\hat{G}(t_0|\mathbf{z}_i)}\right],$$

where $\hat{G}(\cdot|\mathbf{z}_i)$ is the Kaplan–Meier estimator of the conditional censoring distribution given covariates. However, as pointed out in Sect. 3.6.3, it can be assumed that the censoring distribution is independent of the covariates since in a well-designed clinical trial, important prognostic factors are balanced across the treatment groups, featured with administrative censoring.

An alternative approach to constructing an estimating equation is to re-express Eq. (4.45) via the check function defined in Sect. 1.6. Note that given the covariate vector $\mathbf{z}_i$, Eq. (4.45) can be rewritten as

$$\Pr(t_0 < T_i \leq t_0 + \exp(\boldsymbol{\beta}'_{1,\tau|t_0}), \epsilon_i = 1) - \tau\Pr(T_i > t_0) = 0,$$

or equivalently

$$E[I(t_0 < T_i \leq t_0 + \exp(\boldsymbol{\beta}'_{1,\tau|t_0}\mathbf{z}_i), \epsilon_i = 1)] - \tau E[I(T_i > t_0)] = 0,$$

which is also identical to

$$E[I(T_i > t_0)\{\tau - I(T_i \leq t_0 + \exp(\boldsymbol{\beta}'_{1,\tau|t_0}\mathbf{z}_i), \epsilon_i = 1)\}] = 0.$$

Let us define

$$
\begin{aligned}
g_{1,\beta}(T_i) &= I(T_i > t_0)\{\tau - I(T_i \leq t_0 + \exp(\boldsymbol{\beta}'_{1,\tau|t_0}\mathbf{z}_i), \epsilon_i = 1)\} \\
&= I(T_i > t_0)[\tau - I[\log(T_i - t_0) \leq \boldsymbol{\beta}'_{1,\tau|t_0}\mathbf{z}_i, \epsilon_i = 1]] \\
&= I(T_i > t_0)\psi_{1,\tau}(u_i), \quad\quad\quad (4.47)
\end{aligned}
$$

where $u_i = \log(T_i - t_0) - \boldsymbol{\beta}'_{1,\tau|t_0}\mathbf{z}_i$ and

$$\psi_{1,\tau}(u_i) = \tau - I(u_i \leq 0, \epsilon_i = 1),$$

which is the derivative of the check function associated with type 1 events

$$\rho_{1,\tau}(u_i) = u_i[\tau - I(u_i \leq 0, \epsilon_i = 1)].$$

Here note that the check function was defined to include 0 in the upper limit of u_i.

One can notice that, given $\mathbf{z}_i$, it is also true that

$$E[\mathbf{z}_i g_{1,\beta}(T_i)|\mathbf{z}_i] = \int_0^\infty \mathbf{z}_i g_{1,\beta}(T_i)dF_1(T_i|\mathbf{z}_i) = 0,$$

where $F_1(T_i|\mathbf{z}_i]$ is the cumulative incidence function for type 1 events given $\mathbf{z}_i$. Therefore, following the similar arguments as in

Sect. 3.6.3, we can form a score function type estimating equation for type 1 events as

$$\sum_{i=1}^{n} \Delta_{1,i} \mathbf{z}_i I(X_i > t_0)[\tau - I\{X_i \le t_0 + \exp(\boldsymbol{\beta}'_{1,\tau|t_0} \mathbf{z}_i), \epsilon_i = 1\}] = 0,$$

(4.48)

where X_i is the minimum of the potential event time T_i and the potential censoring time C_i, and $\Delta_{1,i}$ is a jump of the pooled cumulative incidence estimates for the distribution of type 1 events.

Lim (2011) showed that the estimate $\hat{\boldsymbol{\beta}}_{1,\tau|t_0}$ from the estimating equation (4.46) is asymptotically consistent and the asymptotic distribution of $n^{-1/2} \mathbf{S}_{1,t_0|\tau,n}(\boldsymbol{\beta}^0_{1,\tau|t_0})$ at the true value of $\boldsymbol{\beta}_{1,\tau|t_0}$, $\boldsymbol{\beta}^0_{1,\tau|t_0}$, is normal with mean zero and a variance–covariance matrix, which can be consistently estimated by $\hat{\boldsymbol{\Gamma}}_{1,\tau|t_0} = n^{-1} \sum_{i=1}^{n} \hat{\boldsymbol{\xi}}_{1,\tau|t_0,i} \hat{\boldsymbol{\xi}}'_{1,\tau|t_0,i}$, where

$$\hat{\boldsymbol{\xi}}_{1,\tau|t_0,i} = \mathbf{z}_i \left[\frac{\left[I\{X_i \le t_0 + \exp(\hat{\boldsymbol{\beta}}'_{1,\tau|t_0} \mathbf{z}_i)\} - I(X_i \le t_0) \right] I(\delta_i = 1)}{\hat{G}(X_i-)} - \tau \frac{I(X_i > t_0)}{\hat{G}(t_0)} \right]$$

$$+ \sum_{l=1}^{n} \left[\mathbf{z}_l \frac{\left[I\{X_l \le t_0 + \exp(\hat{\boldsymbol{\beta}}'_{1,\tau|t_0} \mathbf{z}_l)\} - I(X_l \le t_0) \right] I(\delta_l = 1)}{\hat{G}(X_l-)} \right]$$

$$\times \left[\frac{I(\delta_i = 0) I\{X_i \le t_0 + \exp(\hat{\boldsymbol{\beta}}'_{1,\tau|t_0} \mathbf{z}_l)\}}{\sum_{m=1}^{n} I(X_m \ge X_i)} \right.$$

$$\left. - \sum_{j=1}^{n} \frac{I(\delta_j = 0) I\left[X_j \le \min\{t_0 + \exp(\hat{\boldsymbol{\beta}}'_{1,\tau|t_0} \mathbf{z}_l), X_j\} \right]}{\sum_{m=1}^{n} I(X_m \ge X_j)^2} \right]$$

$$- \sum_{l=1}^{n} \left\{ \mathbf{z}_l \frac{\tau I(X_l > t_0)}{n\hat{G}(t_0)} \right\} \left[\frac{I(\delta_i = 0) I(X_i \le t_0)}{\sum_{m=1}^{n} I(X_m \ge X_i)} - \sum_{j=1}^{n} \frac{I(\delta_j = 0) I\{X_j \le \min(t_0, X_i)\}}{\sum_{m=1}^{n} I(X_m \ge X_j)\}^2} \right].$$

To test the null hypothesis of $H_0 : \boldsymbol{\beta}_{1,\tau|t_0} = \hat{\boldsymbol{\beta}}_{1,\tau|t_0,0}$, a statistic can be constructed as

$$n^{-1} \mathbf{S}'_{1,\tau|t_0,n}(\hat{\boldsymbol{\beta}}_{1,\tau|t_0,0}) \hat{\boldsymbol{\Gamma}}^{-1}_{1,\tau|t_0} \mathbf{S}_{1,\tau|t_0,n}(\hat{\boldsymbol{\beta}}_{1,\tau|t_0,0}),$$

(4.49)

which asymptotically follows a χ^2-distribution with $p + 1$ degrees of freedom. A large observed value of this statistic would result in rejection of the null hypothesis. As for the non-competing risks case discussed in 3.6.3, using the estimating equation itself to form the test statistic would avoid the necessity of estimating the probability density function of type 1 events under competing risks.

Now suppose that we are interested in a local test for a subset of the regression coefficients. Given a partition of the regression coefficients, $\boldsymbol{\beta}_{1,\tau|t_0} = (\boldsymbol{\beta}^{(1)}_{1,\tau|t_0}{}', \boldsymbol{\beta}^{(2)}_{1,\tau|t_0}{}')$, where $\boldsymbol{\beta}^{(1)}_{1,\tau|t_0}$ is an $r \times 1$ vector, let us consider testing the null hypothesis of $H_0 : \boldsymbol{\beta}^{(1)}_{1,\tau|t_0} = \hat{\boldsymbol{\beta}}^{(1)}_{1,\tau|t_0,0}$. One way of eliminating the nuisance parameters $\boldsymbol{\beta}^{(2)}_{1,\tau|t_0}$ would be to form a variation of the minimum dispersion statistic (Basawa and Koul, 1988),

$$
V(\hat{\boldsymbol{\beta}}^{(1)}_{1,\tau|t_0,0}) = \min_{\boldsymbol{\beta}^{(2)}_{1,\tau|t_0}} \{n^{-1}\mathbf{S}_{1,t_0|\tau,n}((\hat{\boldsymbol{\beta}}^{(1)}_{1,\tau|t_0,0}{}', \boldsymbol{\beta}^{(2)}_{1,\tau|t_0}{}')) \, \hat{\Gamma}^{-1}_{1,t_0|\tau}
$$
$$
\mathbf{S}_{1,t_0|\tau,n}((\hat{\boldsymbol{\beta}}^{(1)}_{1,\tau|t_0,0}{}', \boldsymbol{\beta}^{(2)}_{1,\tau|t_0}{}'))\}. \tag{4.50}
$$

Following the arguments in Wei *et al.* (1990, Appendix 2) and Ying *et al.* (1995, Appendix C), it can also be shown that the statistic $V(\hat{\boldsymbol{\beta}}^{(1)}_{1,\tau|t_0,0})$ has approximately a χ^2-distribution with r degrees of freedom (Lim, 2011).

Example 4.6 (Application to NSABP B-04 Dataset). Lim (2011) applied the method developed for the semiparametric quantile residual life regression model under competing risks developed in this section to NSABP B-04 dataset. Competing events were again breast-cancer-related deaths vs. non-breast-cancer-related deaths. Three covariates were included in a multiple regression model, i.e. nodal status, age at diagnosis, and pathological tumor size. Table 4.4, extracted from Lim (2011), summarizes the estimated effects of the covariates on the quantile residual life distribution of breast-cancer-related deaths and associated p-values. As Lim (2011) pointed out, both nodal status and tumor size had negative effects on the quantiles of the residual life distribution of breast-cancer-related deaths at all fixed time points, implying that patients with positive lymph nodes and larger tumor sizes at the diagnosis tend to live shorter than ones with negative lymph

Table 4.4: Regression coefficient estimates ($\hat{\beta}_0$ for the intercept, $\hat{\beta}_1$ for nodal status, $\hat{\beta}_2$ for age, and $\hat{\beta}_3$ for tumor size) and associated p-values for different quantiles (0.1,0.2, and 0.3) at different time points ($t_0 = 0, 2, 4, 6, 8$) (Lim, 2011)

τ	t_0	$\hat{\beta}_0$	p	$\hat{\beta}_1$	p	$\hat{\beta}_2$	p	$\hat{\beta}_3$	p
0.1	1	1.11	<.0001	−0.67	<.0001	0.78	.010	−1.56	<.0001
	2	0.20	.286	−0.41	.296	1.85	.067	−1.89	.008
	4	0.93	.145	−0.44	.103	0.79	.554	−1.49	.147
	6	1.80	<.0001	−1.27	<.0001	0.10	.748	−1.51	.063
	8	2.61	.005	−0.93	.001	−1.51	.289	−0.42	.374
0.2	0	1.02	<.0001	−0.56	<.0001	2.14	.003	−1.63	<.0001
	2	0.74	.004	−0.44	.004	2.49	.007	−1.63	.0003
	4	3.77	<.0001	−0.71	<.0001	−1.89	.838	−2.04	.026
	6	3.54	<.0001	−1.20	<.0001	−1.08	.075	−1.64	.002
	8	6.76	<.0001	−1.07	.005	−5.70	.005	−2.24	.019
0.3	0	1.97	<.0001	−0.77	<.0001	1.75	.0009	−1.81	<.0001
	2	3.18	<.0001	−0.79	<.0001	−0.02	.048	−2.11	<.0001
	4	4.09	<.0001	−1.09	<.0001	−0.92	.189	−1.92	<.0001

nodes and smaller tumor sizes. Interestingly, however, age at diagnosis had positive effects at earlier time points, but the effects go in the other direction at later time points. This might imply that because breast cancers developed in younger patients (possibly genetic effect) are known to be more aggressive, those patients tend to die earlier due to breast cancer recurrence, but patients who have overcome the "high-risk" period (about 2 years) would have longer life expectancy than ones whose diseases were developed at older ages (possibly age effect). In this case, statistical analyses based on a series of quantile residual lifetimes capture a panoramic view of shifting effects of the covariates on the cause-specific quantile residual lifetimes, which could help generating biological or etiological hypotheses.

4.5 Further Reading and Future Direction

Regarding statistical methods for the quantile residual life function for competing risks data, not much other work can be found in the literature. One possible extension of work presented in this chapter would be under the constraint that the sum of the asymptotes of the subdistributions given covariates be 1 (Shi, Cheng, and Jeong, 2013), which is not imposed in the usual parametric and nonparametric competing risks regressions (Fine and Gray, 1999; Jeong and Fine, 2007).

The results may also be extended to a conditional setting. For example, investigators might be interested in inference on the quantile residual lifetime to death conditionally among patients who has recurrence at or beyond a given time point. This case could be viewed as a semi-competing risks setting where a non-terminal event (recurrence) can censor a terminal event (death) but not vice versa (Fine, Jiang, and Chappell, 2001).

Chapter 5

Other Methods for Inference on Quantiles

5.1 Issues in Inference on Quantiles

While the quantiles have many advantages including robustness, straightforward interpretation, and presentation of specific information, they also suffer from some pitfalls. First of all, evaluation of the variance formulas of the quantiles involves estimation of the probability density function under independent and/or dependent censoring, which is often cumbersome. To avoid that hurdle, the minimum dispersion statistics based on an estimating equation as discussed in Chaps. 3 and 4 has been adopted, which, however, produced complicated variance formulas. Second, when the censoring proportion is high, higher quantiles cannot be defined. For example, the censoring proportion is greater than 50%, any quantiles equal to or above the median does not exist, even though investigators might be still interested in those quantities. In this chapter, we review two recent approaches that addressed these issues. The first method is based on the empirical likelihood ratio (ELR), which does not need any variance estimation to infer the quantiles, and the second method is a Bayesian approach that allows nonparametric but stable extrapolation for

J.-H. Jeong, *Statistical Inference on Residual Life*,
Statistics for Biology and Health, DOI 10.1007/978-1-4939-0005-3_5,
© Springer Science+Business Media New York 2014

any non-observable quantiles. For the empirical likelihood approach, we provide a simple example to explain how the method works and then move on to application to the quantile residual life inference. For the Bayesian method, we only provide a brief overview. R codes used in the numerical example are provided in Appendix.

5.2   Empirical Likelihood Approach

The cornerstone for the empirical likelihood-based inference is that the population consists of discrete probability space where the probability mass is assigned to each atom that supports the population. Once an experiment is performed and data are collected, the empirical distribution would reflect the discrete population distribution.

The original concept of the empirical likelihood dates back to Thomas and Grunkemeier (1975), who proposed the likelihood ratio method to estimate the confidence interval for survival probabilities for censored data. Forming the likelihood ratio in their work required estimation of the Kaplan–Meier estimator under the null hypothesis (constrained) by using the Lagrangian multiplier technique. The term "empirical likelihood" was coined by Owen (1988, 1990, 2001) who extended the results from Thomas and Grunkemeier (1975) to the more general settings such as ordinary random sampling models, regression models, autoregressive models. First we review some basics of the empirical likelihood theory presented in Hall and La Scala (1990).

The empirical likelihood method can be mainly used to construct confidence regions of the true parameters. Major advantages of the empirical likelihood method are that (1) confidence regions are not shaped in a predetermined way by forcing symmetry or normality and (2) evaluation of confidence regions via the empirical likelihood requires neither estimation of scale or skewness nor construction of a pivotal statistic.

5.2.1 Empirical Likelihood Ratio for the Population Mean

Let $X_1, X_2, \ldots, X_n$ be a random sample from a population with a parameter θ and $p = (p_1, p_2, \ldots, p_n)$ be a vector of discrete probability masses such that $p_i \geq 0$ and $\sum_{i=1}^{n} p_i = 1$. Suppose $\theta(p)$ is a value assumed by the parameter θ when the population has a discrete probability mass p_i at X_i. This implies that the distribution that X_i's are from is characterized only by a set of probabilities p_i's on X_i's. For example, if θ is the population mean, then $\theta(p) = \sum p_i X_i$. With the random sample of $X_1, X_2, \ldots, X_n$, it will be shown later that $p_i = 1/n$ $(i = 1, 2, \ldots, n)$ maximizes the empirical likelihood function under the general constraint of $\sum_{i=1}^{n} p_i = 1$ to obtain the nonparametric maximum likelihood estimator (MLE) for the population mean.

Now we will investigate the asymptotic distribution of the empirical log-likelihood ratio test statistic to test the null hypothesis of $H_0 : \theta(p) = \mu_0$, where μ_0 is a specified value of the population mean. In general, the empirical likelihood function evaluated at $\theta = \mu_0$ is given by

$$EL(\mu_0) = \max_p \prod_{i=1}^{n} p_i, \text{ subject to } \theta(p) = \mu_0, \sum p_i = 1,$$

so that the ELR can be formed as

$$\mathcal{R}(\mu_0) = \frac{\max_{p:\theta(p)=\mu_0, \sum p_i=1} \prod_{i=1}^{n} p_i}{\max_{p:\sum p_i=1} \prod_{i=1}^{n} p_i}. \tag{5.1}$$

Because both numerator and denominator in (5.1) require maximization subject to constraints, the Lagrangian multiplier technique (Lagrange, 1806) needs to be applied. In the denominator, let us set the objective function to be maximized on a log-scale as $f_1(p) = \sum_{i=1}^{n} \ln(p_i)$ and the constraint as $h(p) = \sum_{i=1}^{n} p_i - 1$. Therefore, to maximize the objective function $f_1(p)$, a Lagrange multiplier λ needs to be determined from the gradient vector equation

$$\frac{df_1(p)}{dp} = \lambda \frac{dh(p)}{dp}. \tag{5.2}$$

By taking the derivative with respect to each p_i, Eq. (5.2) gives the simultaneous equations of $1 - \lambda p_1 = 0$, $1 - \lambda p_2 = 0, \ldots,$ $1 - \lambda p_n = 0$. By summing them up, we have $n - \lambda \sum_{i=1}^{n} p_i = 0$, which gives $\lambda = n$. Thus any i^{th} equation of $1 - \lambda p_i = 0$ ($i = 1, 2, \ldots, n$) gives $p_i = 1/n$. That is, by applying the Lagrange multiplier, the denominator in (5.1) is maximized at $p_i = 1/n$, which gives the nonparametric MLE for the population mean as $\hat{\theta}(p) = \sum_{i=1}^{n} X_i/n$. Therefore, the ELR $\mathcal{R}(\mu_0)$ reduces to

$$\mathcal{R}(\mu_0) = \max_{p:\theta(p)=\mu_0, \sum p_i=1} \prod_{i=1}^{n} (np_i). \tag{5.3}$$

To obtain the complete likelihood ratio, we need to further maximize $f_2(p) = \sum_{i=1}^{n} \ln(np_i)$ with respect to p under an additional constraint

$$g(p) = n(\sum_{i=1}^{n} p_i X_i - \mu_0),$$

where the constant term n has been included for convenience. Now we have the gradient vector equation with two Lagrange multipliers λ and γ as

$$\frac{df_2(p)}{dp} = \lambda \frac{dg(p)}{dp} + \gamma \frac{dh(p)}{dp}. \tag{5.4}$$

By taking the derivative in (5.4) with respect to each p_i, we obtain a set of simultaneous equations of $1 - n\lambda p_1 X_1 - \gamma p_1 = 0$, $1 - n\lambda p_2 X_2 - \gamma p_2 = 0, \ldots, 1 - n\lambda p_n X_n - \gamma p_n = 0$. Summing up both sides of all of these equations gives

$$n - n\lambda \sum_{i=1}^{n} p_i X_i - \gamma \sum_{i=1}^{n} p_i = 0,$$

which leads to $\gamma = n(1 - \lambda\mu_0)$ and hence

$$p_i = \frac{1}{n\{1 + \lambda(X_i - \mu_0)\}}. \tag{5.5}$$

Replacing p_i in $g(p) = \sum_{i=1}^{n} p_i X_i - \mu_0 = \sum_{i=1}^{n} p_i (X_i - \mu_0) = 0$ with (5.5), we have an equation to determine λ as

$$\sum_{i=1}^{n} \left(\frac{1}{1 + \lambda(X_i - \mu_0)} \right) (X_i - \mu_0) = 0. \tag{5.6}$$

Since $\{1 + \lambda(X_i - \mu_0)\}^{-1} \approx 1 - \lambda(X_i - \mu_0)$ asymptotically under the null hypothesis of $H_0 : \theta(p) = \mu_0$ by the binomial expansion, Eq. (5.6) reduces to

$$\sum_{i=1}^{n} \{1 - \lambda(X_i - \mu_0)\}(X_i - \mu_0) \approx 0,$$

which gives $\lambda = (\bar{X} - \mu_0)/S^2$, where $\bar{X} = \sum_{i=1}^{n} X_i/n$ and $S^2 = \sum_{i=1}^{n}(X_i - \mu_0)^2/n$ is the variance of X_i's under the null hypothesis. From (5.3) and (5.5), the empirical log-likelihood is given by

$$l(\mu_0) = -2 \sum_{i=1}^{n} \log(np_i) = 2 \sum_{i=1}^{n} \log\{1 + \lambda(X_i - \mu_0)\},$$

which, by the Taylor series expansion, can be asymptotically approximated by $2\lambda \sum_{i=1}^{n}(X_i - \mu_0) - \lambda^2 \sum_{i=1}^{n}(X_i - \mu_0)^2 = n(\bar{X} - \mu_0)^2/S^2$, which follows asymptotically a chi-square distribution with 1 degree of freedom under the null hypothesis. Thus the asymptotic $100(1 - \alpha)\%$ coverage probability for true μ_0 can be obtained by inverting $P\{l(\mu) \leq \chi^2_{1-\alpha,1}\}$ for μ where $\chi^2_{1-\alpha,1}$ is the $(1 - \alpha)$ percentile of the χ^2-distribution with 1 degree of freedom.

The following theorem modifies the results in (5.5) and (5.6) to a more general case where the weighted probabilities are assigned to the discrete sample space.

Theorem 6 (Zhou, 2005). *Suppose we have a random sample of T_1, T_2,..., T_n (uncensored, UC) from a population with the cumulative distribution function $F(\cdot)$ associated with nonnegative weights $w_1^{(UC)}$, $w_2^{(UC)}$, ..., $w_n^{(UC)}$. The empirical likelihood function based on the weighted random variables is given by $\prod_{i=1}^{n} p_i^{w_i^{(UC)}}$, so that the logarithm of the empirical likelihood function is*

$$\sum_{i=1}^{n} w_i^{(UC)} \log(p_i).$$

The maximization of the above empirical log-likelihood function with respect to p_i subject to two constraints

$$\sum_{i=1}^{n} p_i = 1, \qquad \sum_{i=1}^{n} g(T_i)p_i = \mu_0$$

is given by

$$p_i = \frac{w_i^{(UC)}}{\sum_{j=1}^{n} w_j^{(UC)} + \lambda\{g(T_i) - \mu_0\}}, \tag{5.7}$$

where λ is the solution of the equation

$$\sum_{i=1}^{n} \left(\frac{w_i^{(UC)}\{g(T_i) - \mu_0\}}{\sum_{j=1}^{n} w_j^{(UC)} + \lambda\{g(T_i) - \mu_0\}} \right) = 0. \tag{5.8}$$

As will be exemplified in Sect. 5.2.3, in the above theorem the weight w_i can be the number of tied event times for uncensored observations plus the distributed conditional probabilities that a censored observation would be realized on any of the uncensored observations beyond it.

5.2.2   Kaplan–Meier Estimator; Nonparametric MLE

In Sect. 1.5.4, the martingale representation of the Kaplan–Meier estimator and its asymptotic behavior were reviewed. The empirical likelihood approach for censored data involves nonparametric global maximization of one of the empirical likelihood functions (not under the null hypothesis) by using the fact that the Kaplan–Meier estimator is the nonparametric MLE. In this section, we provide a simple proof of that fact from Kaplan and Meier (1958) as a basis for the ELR for the quantile residual life function to be presented in the next section.

For the right-censored data, suppose that $X_i = \min(T_i, C_i)$ $(i = 1, 2, \ldots, n)$ is a random variable for observed survival time and $S(t)$ is the survival function for T. Excluding observed censoring times, suppose that $t_{(1)}, t_{(2)}, \ldots$ and $t_{(k)}$ are ordered failure times. It is convenient to partition the entire time interval as $0 = t_{(0)} < t_{(1)} < t_{(2)} < \ldots < t_{(k)} < t_{(k+1)} = \infty$ to present conditional arguments in terms of number of failures and number of subjects at risk. Define d_j and c_j to be the number of failures at $t_{(j)}$ $(j = 1, 2, \ldots, k)$ and the number of censored events within a half-closed interval $[t_{(j)}, t_{(j+1)})$, respectively. Assuming that the nonparametric MLE would assign 0 probabilities between failure times, the likelihood function takes a form of

$$
\begin{aligned}
L &= \prod_{j=1}^{k} \{S(t_{(j-1)}) - S(t_{(j)})\}^{d_j} S(t_{(j)})^{c_j} \\
&= \prod_{j=1}^{k} \{1 - S(t_{(j)})/S(t_{(j-1)})\}^{d_j} S(t_{(j-1)})^{d_j} S(t_{(j)})^{c_j}. \quad (5.9)
\end{aligned}
$$

Note that this is a nonparametric version of the likelihood function, or the empirical likelihood, in that the probability mass at each failure time is expressed as a jump of the discrete survival function and any censoring time that occurred between $t_{(j)}$ and just prior to $t_{(j+1)}$ is assumed to have been censored at $t_{(j)}$.

Because the conditional probability of surviving from $t_{(j-1)}$ to $t_{(j)}$ is given by $P(T > t_{(j)}|T > t_{(j-1)}) = S(t_{(j)})/S(t_{(j-1)}) \equiv \pi_j$, we have $S(t_{(j)}) = \pi_1 \pi_2 \ldots \pi_j$. Therefore the likelihood function (5.9) becomes

$$
L = \prod_{j=1}^{k} (1 - \pi_j)^{d_j} (\pi_1 \pi_2 \ldots \pi_{j-1})^{d_j + c_j} \pi_j^{c_j}, \quad (5.10)
$$

Defining $\pi_0 = 1$, the likelihood function (5.10) can be rewritten as

$$
\begin{aligned}
L &= \left[(1 - \pi_1)^{d_1} \pi_0^{d_1 + c_1} \pi_1^{c_1} \right] \left[(1 - \pi_2)^{d_2} \pi_1^{d_2 + c_2} \pi_2^{c_2} \right] \\
&\quad \times \left[(1 - \pi_3)^{d_3} (\pi_1 \pi_2)^{d_3 + c_3} \pi_3^{c_3} \right] \cdots \\
&= (1 - \pi_1)^{d_1} \pi_1^{c_1 + \sum_{l=2}^{k}(d_l + c_l)} (1 - \pi_2)^{d_2} \pi_2^{c_2 + \sum_{l=3}^{k}(d_l + c_l)} \\
&\quad \times (1 - \pi_3)^{d_3} \pi_3^{c_3 + \sum_{l=4}^{k}(d_l + c_l)} \cdots \\
&= \prod_{j=1}^{k} (1 - \pi_j)^{d_j} \pi_j^{r_j - d_j}, \quad (5.11)
\end{aligned}
$$

where $r_j = \sum_{l \geq j}(d_l + c_l)$. Taking the first derivative of the logarithm of the likelihood function (5.11) and setting it to 0 gives the maximum likelihood equation

$$
\sum_{j=1}^{k} \left[\frac{r_j(1 - \pi_j) - d_j}{\pi_j(1 - \pi_j)} \right] = 0,
$$

which implies that for all j,

$$\frac{r_j(1 - \pi_j) - d_j}{\pi_j(1 - \pi_j)} = 0.$$

From this, we obtain the MLE for π_j as $\hat{\pi}_j = 1 - d_j/r_j$. By using the invariance property of the MLE, the nonparametric MLE for $S(t_{(j)})$ is given by

$$\hat{S}(t_{(j)}) = \prod_{l=1}^{j} (1 - d_l/r_l),$$

or, in general

$$\hat{S}(t) = \prod_{t_{(j)} \leq t} (1 - d_j/r_j), \tag{5.12}$$

which is the product-limit, or Kaplan–Meier, estimator.

From (5.12), note that a jump of the Kaplan–Meier estimator at each ordered uncensored observation $t_{(j)}$ $(j = 1, 2, \ldots, k)$ can be expressed as $k_{(1)} = 1/n$ and

$$k_{(j)} = \left(\frac{d_j}{r_j}\right) \prod_{l=1}^{j-1} \left(1 - \frac{d_l}{r_l}\right), \quad j = 2, \ldots, k.$$

By using all the indicator functions for both uncensored and censored observations $\delta_{(i)}$ $(i = 1, 2, \ldots, n)$ corresponding to ordered observations $x_{(i)}$, $k_{(j)}$ can be equivalently expressed as (Stute, 1996) $\Delta_1 = \delta_{(1)}/n$ and

$$\begin{aligned}
\Delta_i &= \left\{\frac{\delta_{(i)}}{n - (i-1)}\right\} \prod_{l=1}^{i-1} \left\{1 - \frac{1}{n - (l-1)}\right\}^{\delta_{(l)}} \\
&= \frac{\delta_{(i)}}{n - i + 1} \prod_{l=1}^{i-1} \left(\frac{n-l}{n-l+1}\right)^{\delta_{(l)}}, \quad i = 2, \ldots, n. \tag{5.13}
\end{aligned}$$

Zhou *et al.* (2012) interestingly showed that the jumps of the Kaplan–Meier estimator are closely related to the inverse probability weighted censoring (IPWC) estimator of Laan and Robins (2003) and Rotnitzky and Robins (2005). Specifically under the independence assumption between T and C, we have $\Pr(X > t) = \Pr(T > t)\Pr(C > t)$, which empirically implies that

$$1 - \hat{H}(t) = [1 - \hat{F}(t)][1 - \hat{G}(t)], \qquad (5.14)$$

where $\hat{H}(t)$ is the empirical cumulative distribution based on X_i, and $\hat{F}(t)$ and $\hat{G}(t)$ are the estimated cumulative probabilities from the Kaplan–Meier estimators for T_i based on (X_i, δ_i) and for C_i based on $(X_i, 1 - \delta_i)$, respectively. Consider the increments of both sides in (5.14) when $t = X_i$ with $\delta_i = 1$. Because the term $1 - \hat{G}(t)$ is constant when $\delta_i = 1$, we have

$$d[1 - \hat{H}(t)] = [1 - \hat{G}(t)]d[1 - \hat{F}(t)],$$

which gives $1/n = k_i[1 - \hat{G}(X_i)]$, so that a jump of the Kaplan–Meier can also be expressed as k_i^*/n, where

$$k_i^* = \frac{\delta_i}{1 - \hat{G}_{KM}(X_i)},$$

which is the IPWC estimator.

5.2.3 Constrained EM Algorithm for Censored Data

In Sect. 5.2.1, we have demonstrated that the Lagrangian multiplier technique could be applied to maximize the empirical likelihood functions for the population mean (uncensored) under the constraints. However, application of the Lagrangian multiplier is not straightforward for censored data as illustrated in the following example.

Example 5.1. (Zhou, 2005): Suppose that $T_1, T_2, \ldots T_n$ is a random sample from the population with the cumulative distribution function $F(\cdot)$ subject to right censoring, so that we observe $X_i = \min(T_i, C_i)$ and $\delta_i = I(T_i \le C_i)$, where C_i's are the potential censoring times.

In the light of the nonparametric likelihood function given in (5.9), the empirical likelihood function for censored data can generally be expressed as

$$EL(p) = \prod_{i=1}^{n} \{p_i\}^{\delta_i} \{ \sum_{X_j > X_i} p_j \}^{1-\delta_i}, \tag{5.15}$$

where $0 \leq p_i$ for $1 \leq i \leq n$ and $\sum p_i = 1$, so that the logarithm of the empirical likelihood function is given by

$$\log(EL(p)) = \sum_{i=1}^{n} \left\{ \delta_i \log(p_i) + (1 - \delta_i) \log \left(\sum_{X_j > X_i} p_i \right) \right\}.$$

As in Sect. 5.2.1, let us consider the maximization of the above log-likelihood function with the constraints of $\sum_{i=1}^{n} p_i X_i = \mu_0$ and $\sum_{i=1}^{n} p_i = 1$ under the null hypothesis of $H_0 : \text{mean}(F) \equiv \theta = \mu_0$. An immediate application of the Lagrangian multipliers λ and γ yields the following equation: for each i,

$$\frac{\delta_i}{p_i} + \sum_{k=1}^{n} (1 - \delta_k) \frac{I(X_k < X_i)}{\sum_{X_j > X_k} p_j} - \lambda X_i - \gamma,$$

which does not have a simple solution for p_i. Maximization of the empirical likelihood function under the general form of the mean type constraint $\int g(t) dF(t) = \mu_0$ would have the similar difficulty.

To overcome this hurdle, Zhou (2005) modified the constrained EM algorithm (Turnbull, 1976) and applied it to the empirical likelihood inference for censored data. The modified constrained EM is described below.

E-Step: Given the cumulative distribution function F, the weight, w_j, at an uncensored observation t_j is evaluated from

$$w_j = \sum_{i=1}^{n} E_F \{I(T_i = t_j) | X_i, \delta_i\}.$$

Specifically, first we determine the initial weight on each uncensored observation t_j's as $E_F\{I(T_i = t_j) | X_i, \delta_i\} = \Pr(T_i = t_j | X_i =$

$T_i, \delta_i = 1) = 1$ and the value of $w_j = 2$, for example, would imply that there are two uncensored observations tied at t_j. For a censored observation X_i, it is known that the true failure time T_i should be greater than X_i and furthermore it could be one of the uncensored observations beyond that censoring time, given the realized data. Given that $X_i = C_i$ and $\delta_i = 0$, we have $\Pr(T_i = t_j | X_i = C_i, \delta_i = 0) = \Pr(T_i = t_j | T_i > X_i) = \Pr(T_i = t_j)/\Pr(T_i > X_i) = dF(t_j)/\{1 - F(X_i)\}$ for $t_j > X_i$. This implies that the conditional probability of $T_i = t_j$ given $T_i > X_i$, i.e. $dF(t_j)/\{1 - F(X_i)\}$, needs to be added to all of the initial weights for t_j beyond X_i (See Example 5.2 for more details). This weighting scheme attempts to recover the effect of censored observations by assigning an additional weight to *each uncensored* (case-wise) observation given the data, rather than synthesizing the data (Koul *et al.*, 1981) or necessitating iterative calculation of the estimator (Buckley and James, 1979). This step is identical to the E-Step of Turnbull (1976) and produces pseudo observations $X_j = t_j$ and associated weights w_j.

M-Step: With the values of (t_j, w_j) $(j = 1, 2, \ldots, k)$ from the E-Step, determine p_i's by using the formulas (5.7) and (5.8), which would be a new estimate of the cumulative distribution function.

These EM steps need to be iterated until convergence. The convergence criterion can be set in such a way that the iteration stops when the values of the log-empirical likelihood no longer increase. Zhou (2005) showed that the solution of this EM algorithm is equivalent to the constrained maximization of the log-likelihood function. A reasonable set of the starting values for the EM algorithm would be the nonparametric maximum likelihood estimates such as the Kaplan–Meier estimates. Zhou (2005) also considered the case of left-truncated and right-censored data.

Example 5.2. In this example, first we are interested in calculating the empirical likelihood function under the null hypothesis of $H_0 : \theta(p) = \sum_{j=1}^{k} g(t_j) p_j = \mu_0$, where k is the number of distinct uncensored observations t_j's. For simplicity, we take $g(t_j) = t_j$.

Suppose we have the original observed data

$$x^{(0)} = (x_1^{(0)}, x_2^{(0)}, \ldots, x_{12}^{(0)}) = (1, 1, 1.5, 2, 2, 3, 4, 4, 4.5, 5, 5, 6)$$

and

$$\delta^{(0)} = (\delta_1^{(0)}, \delta_2^{(0)}, \ldots, \delta_{12}^{(0)}) = (1, 0, 1, 0, 0, 1, 0, 1, 1, 1, 1, 1).$$

Note that there are two tied censored observations at $x_4^{(0)} = x_5^{(0)} = 2.0$ and two tied uncensored observations at $x_{10}^{(0)} = x_{11}^{(0)} = 5.0$. Figure 5.1 graphically displays the mock dataset ordered in length, where "x" and "o" imply uncensored and censored observations, respectively.

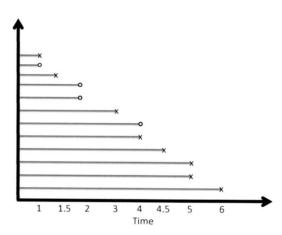

Fig. 5.1: A mock dataset ordered in length

After eliminating each of the same kind of the tied observations, we have

$$x = (x_1, x_2, \ldots, x_{10}) = (1, 1, 1.5, 2, 3, 4, 4, 4.5, 5, 6)$$

and

$$\delta = (\delta_1, \delta_2, \ldots, \delta_{10}) = (1, 0, 1, 0, 1, 0, 1, 1, 1, 1), \tag{5.16}$$

with the initial weights

$$w = (w_1, w_2, \ldots, w_{10}) = (1, 1, 1, 2, 1, 1, 1, 1, 2, 1).$$

Therefore only for the uncensored (UC) observations

$$t = (t_1, t_2, \ldots, t_7) = (1, 1.5, 3, 4, 4.5, 5, 6)$$

the initial weights are given by

$$w^{(UC)} = (w_1^{(UC)}, w_2^{(UC)}, \ldots, w_7^{(UC)}) = (1, 1, 1, 1, 1, 2, 1).$$

Now for each censored observation x_i ($i = 2, 4, 6$), we need to calculate the conditional probability of $dF(t_j)/\{1 - F(x_i)\}$ for $t_j > x_i$ and add it to the initial weights $w_j^{(UC)}$'s beyond x_i. Here $dF(t_j)$ can be replaced by the weighted point probability mass at t_j, denoted as p_j, and $1 - F(x_i)$ can be replaced by the partial sum of the weighted point probability masses beyond x_i, denoted as $S(x_i)$, under the null hypothesis. Since the indicator vector (5.16) indicates that the second, fourth, and sixth observations are censored, the weights adjusted for the censored observations are given by

$$
\begin{aligned}
w^{(adj)} &= (w_1^{(adj)}, w_2^{(adj)}, \ldots, w_7^{(adj)}) \\
&= \Big(1, 1 + \frac{p_2}{S(x_2)}, 1 + \frac{p_3}{S(x_2)} + \frac{2p_3}{S(x_4)}, 1 + \frac{p_4}{S(x_2)} + \frac{2p_4}{S(x_4)}, \\
&\qquad 1 + \frac{p_5}{S(x_2)} + \frac{2p_5}{S(x_4)} + \frac{p_5}{S(x_6)}, 2 + \frac{p_6}{S(x_2)} + \frac{2p_6}{S(x_4)} + \frac{p_6}{S(x_6)}, \\
&\qquad 1 + \frac{p_7}{S(x_2)} + \frac{2p_7}{S(x_4)} + \frac{p_7}{S(x_6)} \Big),
\end{aligned}
$$

where $S(x_2) = \sum_{j=2}^{7} p_j$, $S(x_4) = \sum_{j=3}^{7} p_j$, and $S(x_6) = \sum_{j=5}^{7} p_j$. Note that two censored observations tied at 2 were weighted accordingly.

One step estimates for p_j and hence $S(x_i)$ ($i = 2, 4, 6$) can be achieved by plugging t_j ($j = 1, 2, \ldots, 7$) and $w_j^{(UC)}$ ($j = 1, 2, \ldots, 7$) into (5.7) and (5.8). By setting $\mu_0 = 3.5$, we obtain

$$
\begin{aligned}
\hat{p} &= (\hat{p}_1, \hat{p}_2, \ldots, \hat{p}_7) \\
&= (0.159, 0.151, 0.131, 0.120, 0.115, 0.222, 0.103),
\end{aligned}
$$

and hence

$$\hat{S}(x_2) = 0.841, \quad \hat{S}(x_4) = 0.690, \quad \hat{S}(x_6) = 0.440,$$

so that the adjusted weights can be estimated as

$$\hat{w}^{(adj)} = (1.0, 1.179, 1.534, 1.490, 1.733, 3.409, 1.655).$$

After repeating this procedure until convergence, we obtain the final estimates of the empirical distribution as

$$\hat{p}^{final} = (0.149, 0.152, 0.145, 0.111, 0.128, 0.225, 0.091),$$

and hence

$$\hat{S}(x_2) = 0.851, \quad \hat{S}(x_4) = 0.70, \quad \hat{S}(x_6) = 0.444.$$

Finally the log-empirical likelihood function under the null hypothesis can be evaluated as

$$
\begin{aligned}
\log EL_{H_0} &= \log(EL(\hat{p}^{final})) \\
&= \sum_{j=1}^{7} \left\{ \delta_j^{(UC)} \log(\hat{p}_j^{final}) \right\} + \sum_{i=2,4,6} \left\{ \delta_i^{(C)} \log(\hat{S}(x_i)) \right\} = -17.05,
\end{aligned}
$$

where $\delta^{(UC)} = (1, 1, 1, 1, 1, 2, 1)$ and $\delta^{(C)} = \left(\delta_2^{(C)}, \delta_4^{(C)}, \delta_6^{(C)} \right) = (1, 2, 1)$.

Evaluation of the log-empirical likelihood under the general constraint $\sum_{j=1}^{k} p_j = 1$ is straightforward. In Sect. 5.2.2, we have shown that the Kaplan–Meier would be the nonparametric MLE that maximizes the empirical log-likelihood function. Table 5.1 summarizes the weighted Kaplan–Meier (WKM) estimates together with the estimated jumps $(\hat{p}_i)$ based on (x_i, δ_i, w_i) $(i = 1, 2, \ldots, 10)$ in (5.16). The WKM estimates were calculated from

$$\hat{S}_{WKM}(t) = \prod_{x_{(i)} \le t} \left(1 - w_i \frac{d_i}{r_i} \right).$$

Therefore the log-empirical likelihood function under the general constraint of $\sum_{i=1}^{k} p_i = 1$ can be evaluated as

$$\log EL_{general} = \sum_{i:\delta_i=1} w_i \log(\hat{p}_i) + \sum_{i:\delta_i=0} w_i \log\{\hat{S}_{WKM}(x_i)\} = -16.43,$$

so that the empirical log-likelihood ratio is given by $2(\log EL_{general} - \log EL_{H_0}) = 2(-16.43 + 17.05) = 1.24$, which gives the p-value of 0.26 under the χ^2 distribution with 1 degree of freedom. This implies that the null hypothesis $H_0 : \theta(p) = 3.5$ cannot be rejected at the significance level of 0.05.

R codes used to generate the dataset and to perform data analysis presented in this example are provided in Appendix A.6.

Table 5.1: Estimation of the jumps of the WKM as the empirical probability masses under the general constraint of $\sum_{i=1}^{k} p_i = 1$

X_i	δ_i	w_i	$\hat{S}_{WKM}(X_i)$	Jumps $(\hat{p}_i)$
1.0	1	1	0.9166667	0.08333333
1.0	0	1	0.9166667	0.00000000
1.5	1	1	0.8250000	0.09166667
2.0	0	2	0.8250000	0.00000000
3.0	1	1	0.7071429	0.11785714
4.0	1	1	0.5892857	0.11785714
4.0	0	1	0.5892857	0.00000000
4.5	1	1	0.4419643	0.14732143
5.0	1	2	0.1473214	0.29464286
6.0	1	1	0.0000000	0.14732143

5.2.4 Estimating Equation for Quantile Residual Life

As defined in Chap. 3, the τ-quantile residual life function is the τ-percentile of the distribution of the residual lifetimes $T - t_0$ at time t_0 given $T > t_0$. In this section, we express the estimating equation for the τ-quantile residual life function in terms of the check function, which will be used as the constraint under the null hypothesis in the ELR (Zhou and Jeong, 2011). The τ-quantile residual life function q at time t_0 can be defined from the cumulative distribution function of the residual life distribution

$$\Pr(T - t_0 \leq q | T > t_0) = \tau,$$

which is equivalent to

$$F(t_0 + q) - (1 - \tau)F(t_0) - \tau = 0, \tag{5.17}$$

where $F(t) = \Pr(T \leq t)$ is the cumulative distribution function of the random variable T. Once the data are observed, the cumulative distribution function $F(t)$ can be replaced by the empirical distribution function $\hat{F}_n(t)$ to estimate q.

Or equivalently, we can consider the equation

$$H_0 : E[g_q(T)] = \int_0^\infty g_q(t)dF(t) = 0, \tag{5.18}$$

where

$$g_q(t) = I[(T - t_0) \le q] - (1 - \tau)I(T \le t_0) - \tau.$$

From (5.18), the estimating equation for the τ-th quantile residual life q is given by

$$\int g_q(t)d\hat{F}_n(t) = 0, \tag{5.19}$$

where $\hat{F}_n(t)$ denotes the empirical distribution function without censoring. For censored data with $X_i = \min(T_i, C_i)$ and $\delta_i = I(T_i \le C_i)$, however, the empirical distribution $\hat{F}_n(t)$ needs to be replaced with the Kaplan–Meier estimator $\hat{F}_{KM}(t)$. Therefore the estimating Eq. (5.19) becomes

$$\sum_{i=1}^n \Delta_i g_q(X_i) = 0, \tag{5.20}$$

where Δ_i is the probability mass that $\hat{F}_{KM}(t)$ assigns on (X_i, δ_i), defined in (5.13).

The estimating equation in (5.20) can be expressed as the derivative of the check function defined in Sect. 1.6. Note that the function $g_q(t)$ in (5.18) at X_i can be written as

$$\begin{aligned}
g_q(X_i) &= I[(X_i - t_0) \le q] - (1 - \tau)I[X_i \le t_0] - \tau \\
&= \tau I(X_i > t_0) + I((X_i - t_0) \le q) - I(X_i - t_0 \le 0) \\
&= I(X_i > t_0)[\tau - I((X_i - t_0) \le q)], \tag{5.21}
\end{aligned}$$

because the event $I((X_i - t_0) \le q) - I(X_i - t_0 \le 0)$ is equivalent to $I(0 < X_i - t_0 \le q)$ and hence to $I(X_i - t_0 > 0)I(X_i - t_0 \le q)$. Therefore the estimating Eq. (5.20) can be expressed as

$$\sum_{i=1}^n \Delta_i I[X_i > t_0]\psi_\tau((X_i - t_0) - q) = 0, \tag{5.22}$$

or equivalently as a minimization problem of

$$\min_q \sum_{i=1}^{n} \Delta_i I[X_i > t_0] \rho_\tau ((X_i - t_0) - q).$$

Note that in Example 5.2 the function $g(t)$ and μ_0 can be replaced by $g_q(t)$ in (5.21) and 0, respectively, to evaluate the ELR for testing the quantile residual life in one-sample case. Zhou and Jeong (2012) further extended it to the two-sample case. R package `emplik` has been developed by Zhou (2005), which includes the procedures `el.cen.EM` and `el.cen.EM2`. The utility of the procedure `el.cen.EM2` was demonstrated in Zhou and Jeong (2012) to numerically calculate the ELR statistic and confidence intervals for the mean and median residual lifetimes for censored survival data.

5.2.5 Empirical Likelihood Inference on Quantile Residual Life Regression

As discussed in Sect. 3.6, we consider an accelerated failure time (AFT) model (Cox and Oakes, 1984) that regresses potential confounding factors (covariates, $\mathbf{z}_i$) on the residual lifetimes on a log-scale at a fixed time point t_0.

Suppose n independent and identically distributed random variables $(T_i, \mathbf{z}_i)$ $(i = 1, 2, \ldots, n)$ are generated from the true model subject to error ϵ_i

$$\tau - \text{quantile}\{\log(T_i - t_0) | T_i > t_0, \mathbf{z}_i\} = \boldsymbol{\beta}' \mathbf{z}_i + \epsilon_i, \qquad (5.23)$$

where $'$ denotes a transpose of a vector and $\boldsymbol{\beta} = \boldsymbol{\beta}_{\tau|t_0}$ represents the τ-quantile-specific covariate effects on the residual lifetimes at t_0. The dependency of the covariate effects on the follow-up time t_0 distinguishes the proposed *residual* quantile residual life regression from the regular quantile regression. The model implicitly assumes that the conditional quantile of the residual life distribution on a log-scale $(= \log(T_i - t_0))$ is a linear function of the given covariates $(= \boldsymbol{\beta}' \mathbf{z}_i)$. Testing the null hypothesis of $H_0 : \boldsymbol{\beta} = \boldsymbol{\beta}_0$ would imply to test any specific linear relationship with the slope of $\boldsymbol{\beta}_0$ between the quantiles of $\log(T_i - t_0)$ ($i = 1, 2, \ldots, n$) and the covariate vector $\mathbf{z}_i$.

For the right-censored data, we observe $(X_i, \delta_i, \mathbf{z}_i)$ ($i = 1, 2, \ldots, n$) where $X_i = \min(T_i, C_i)$, $\delta_i = I(T_i \leq C_i)$. From (3.39), the estimating equation for the regression parameters under the model (5.23) is given by

$$\sum_{i=1}^{n} \Delta_i I[X_i > t_0] \mathbf{z}_i \psi_\tau (\log(X_i - t_0) - \boldsymbol{\beta}' \mathbf{z}_i) = 0, \qquad (5.24)$$

where Δ_i is a jump of the Kaplan–Meier estimates based on (X_i, δ_i) defined in (5.13). Note that this estimating equation provides a weighted quantile regression estimator for the residual life distribution under censoring and reduces to the estimating equation used by Jung *et al.* (2009) with $\Delta_i = 1$ for all i when there is no censoring. When there is censoring, the two estimating equations use slightly different weighting schemes, but both methods provide consistent estimates (Jung *et al.*, 2009; Kim *et al.*, 2012).

Now let us consider the ELR under the model (5.23)

$$\mathcal{R}(\boldsymbol{\beta}) = \frac{\max_{p:\sum_{i=i}^{n} p_i=1, \sum_{i=1}^{n} p_i g_\beta(X_i-t_0)=0} EL(p)}{\max_{p:\sum_{i=1}^{n} p_i=1} EL(p)}, \qquad (5.25)$$

where

$$EL(p) = \prod_{i=1}^{n} \{p_i\}^{\delta_i} \{ \sum_{X_j > X_i} p_j \}^{1-\delta_i},$$

and

$$g_\beta(X_i - t_0) = I[X_i > t_0] \mathbf{z}_i \psi_\tau (\log(X_i - t_0) - \boldsymbol{\beta}' \mathbf{z}_i).$$

As shown in Sect. 5.2.2, the jumps of the Kaplan–Meier estimates, $\Delta_{KM} = (\Delta_1, \Delta_2, \ldots, \Delta_n)$, based on (X_i, δ_i) in (5.13) maximize the denominator of the ELR $\mathcal{R}(\boldsymbol{\beta})$. Accordingly the ELR in (5.25) under the null hypothesis of $H_0 : \boldsymbol{\beta} = \boldsymbol{\beta}_0$ can be expressed as

$$\mathcal{R}(\boldsymbol{\beta}_0) = \frac{EL(\hat{p}_0|\boldsymbol{\beta}_0)}{EL(\Delta_{KM})}, \qquad (5.26)$$

where $\hat{p}_0$ is the estimates of p that maximizes $EL(p)$ under the constraint of

$$\sum_{i=1}^{n} p_i g_\beta(X_i - t_0) = 0, \tag{5.27}$$

and $EL(\hat{p}_0|\boldsymbol{\beta}_0)$ and $EL(\Delta_{KM})$ are the empirical likelihood functions evaluated at $\hat{p}_0$ and at Δ_{KM}, respectively.

Under some regularity conditions and if $\boldsymbol{\beta}_0$ denotes a vector of the null values of $\boldsymbol{\beta}$ in r dimension, it can be proven that $-2 \log R(\boldsymbol{\beta}_0)$ is asymptotically χ^2-distributed with r degrees of freedom (Kim $et\ al.$, 2012). A $100(1 - \alpha)\%$ confidence interval or region can be also constructed by inverting the likelihood ratio, i.e., $\{\boldsymbol{\beta} : -2 \log \mathcal{R}(\boldsymbol{\beta}) \leq \chi^2_{1-\alpha,r}\}$ where $\chi^2_{1-\alpha,r}$ is the $(1 - \alpha)^{th}$ quantile of a χ^2 distribution with r degrees of freedom. Note that the constraint Eq. (5.27) is equivalent to the estimating Eq. (5.24) when p_i's in the constraint equation are replaced by Δ_i's.

In many applications, only a subset of the vector $\boldsymbol{\beta}$ is of interest. If we have a partition of $\boldsymbol{\beta} = (\boldsymbol{\beta}_1, \boldsymbol{\beta}_2)$ and only $\boldsymbol{\beta}_1$ is of interest, the profile likelihood ratio can be constructed as $\sup_{\boldsymbol{\beta}_2} \mathcal{R}(\boldsymbol{\beta}_1, \boldsymbol{\beta}_2)$. If $\boldsymbol{\beta}_{10}$ denotes the null value of $\boldsymbol{\beta}_1$ in r_1 dimension, it can also be proven that $-2 \log \sup_{\boldsymbol{\beta}_2} \mathcal{R}(\boldsymbol{\beta}_{10}, \boldsymbol{\beta}_2)$ follows asymptotically a χ^2 distribution with r_1 degrees of freedom (Kim $et\ al.$, 2012).

Extending the computational procedure of the constrained EM algorithm to this quantile residual life regression only requires to replace the g-function $g(T_i)$ and μ_0 in (5.7) and (5.8) with $g_\beta(t_j - t_0)$ and $\boldsymbol{\beta}_0$, respectively, where t_j is an uncensored observation.

5.3 Bayesian Inference Under Heavy Censoring

As briefly mentioned in Sect. 5.1, higher quantiles might not be able to be nonparametrically estimated under heavy censoring. For example, the median cannot be estimated nonparametrically unless the estimated Kaplan–Meier curve reaches 0.5. Frequentist and Bayesian parametric methods could be adopted for the purpose, but it is well known that the parametric approaches might suffer from violation of strong underlying assumption unless it is correctly specified. These difficulties seem to have motivated development of a series of nonparametric Bayesian approaches in the literature, which allow for flexible and adaptive modeling of the unknown failure time distribution via a Dirichlet process (DP) mixture (Ferguson, 1973, 1974). For example, Kottas and Gelfand (2001) developed nonparametric Bayesian methods to model the error distribution of the log-transformed survival times, which Gelfand and Kottas (2003) applied to inference on the median residual lifetimes under the AFT model. As pointed out by Ishwaran and James (2001) and Gelfand and Kottas (2002), in the Bayesian nonparametric methods developed up to that point, the DP mixture models were fitted by marginalizing over a DP mixture prior, resulting in the Pólya urn Gibbs sampler (Escobar, 1994; Escobar and West, 1995), which does not allow for direct inference on the general functionals of the DP mixture model such as the survival function and hazard function. Later Kottas (2006) provided a method to approximate the general functions associated with survival data by extending Gelfand and Kottas (2002).

For inference on the quantile residual life, Park, Jeong, and Lee (2012) recently proposed the blocked Gibbs sampler (Ishwaran and James, 2001) to fit the Weibull DP mixture model for the unknown failure time distribution, which allows for direct posterior inference on the general functionals of the DP mixture model. They also exploited partial collapse (van Dyk and Park, 2008) to improve the convergence of the blocked Gibbs sampler. They applied the proposed procedure to a dataset from a clinical trial on breast cancer, which consisted of two comparison groups, placebo and tamoxifen. Figure 5.2 compares the Kaplan–Meier (solid line) and nonparametric Bayesian estimates (dashed line) for the tamoxifen group at the origin, i.e. $t_0 = 0$. Since the estimated Kaplan–Meier curve does not reach 0.5, the median failure time cannot be estimated nonparametrically. However, the survival curve estimated from the nonparametric Bayesian method gives almost identical estimates up to the last observed failure, but extrapolates further even though 95 % credible intervals (dotted lines) become wider toward the tail of the distribution as the level of uncertainty increases.

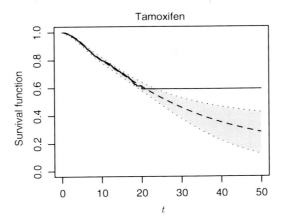

Fig. 5.2: Comparison of Kaplan–Meier and nonparametric Bayesian estimates in a treatment group from a breast cancer study (Park *et al.*, 2012, *Statistics in Medicine*)

5.4   Further Reading and Future Direction

The book by Owen (2001) would be an excellent reference for the empirical likelihood theory and application. Not much work can be found in the topic of empirical likelihood inference and quantile residual life combined. As mentioned in Sect. 3.7, Kim and Yang (2011) extended the quantile regression model to a clustered response case, but without censoring. Further extension of their work to a regression model for quantile residual life with censoring might be of interest. Also the results presented in this chapter might be extended to the (semi)competing risks setting even though a stronger assumption may be needed.

Chapter 6

Study Design Based on Quantile (Residual Life)

Statistical design of a time-to-event study is usually based on the log-rank test, which is optimal for the proportional hazards model to test for the hazard ratio. However, it would be more straightforward to design a study to test for a difference in quantile (residual) lifetimes, say to detect a difference in the median residual lifetime due to a drug effect. In this chapter, we consider such design strategies both in the absence and in the presence of competing risks. First for the non-competing risks case, we derive the sample size formula based on the difference in two quantile residual lifetimes, assuming exponential distributions for event and censoring distributions, which is compared with one derived from the log-rank test statistic that uses the hazard ratio. For the competing risks case, the sample size formula is derived from the cause-specific parameterization discussed in Sect. 4.3.1.

J.-H. Jeong, *Statistical Inference on Residual Life*,
Statistics for Biology and Health, DOI 10.1007/978-1-4939-0005-3_6,
© Springer Science+Business Media New York 2014

6.1   Sample Size Calculation in the Absence of Competing Risks

Let us define $q_k = \theta_{t_0}^{(k)}(\tau; \boldsymbol{\psi}^{(k)})$ to be the τ-quantile from a residual life distribution for group k ($k = 1, 2$) at time t_0 and $V_k = \mathrm{Var}(\hat{q}_k)$, where $\hat{q}_k = \theta_{t_0}^{(k)}(\tau; \widehat{\boldsymbol{\psi}}^{(k)})$. Under the null hypothesis $H_0 : \Delta = q_1 - q_2 = 0$, the two-sample statistic proposed in Sect. 3.4.2, $W_{t_0}(\tau) = (\hat{q}_1 - \hat{q}_2)/\sqrt{V_1 + V_2}$, can be used to derive the sample size formula. For a two-sided test with type I error probability of α, to detect a τ-quantile residual life difference $\Delta = \Delta_1$, the power function $\pi_\alpha(\tau)$ can be defined as

$$\pi_\alpha(\tau) = \Pr(W_{t_0}(\tau) \geq z_{1-\frac{\alpha}{2}} | \Delta = \Delta_1), \qquad (6.1)$$

where $z_{1-\frac{\alpha}{2}}$ is the $(1 - \frac{\alpha}{2})$th percentile of the standard normal distribution. Denoting β for type II error probability, the power function (6.1) can be further specified as

$$\pi_\alpha(\tau) = \Pr\left(\frac{\hat{q}_1 - \hat{q}_2 - \Delta_1}{\sqrt{V_1 + V_2}} \geq z_{1-\frac{\alpha}{2}} - \frac{\Delta_1}{\sqrt{V_1 + V_2}} \right) = 1 - \beta,$$

implying that

$$z_{1-\frac{\alpha}{2}} - \frac{\Delta_1}{\sqrt{V_1 + V_2}} = z_\beta. \qquad (6.2)$$

As a specific example, let us consider the exponential distribution to design a study with time-to-event outcome. Suppose that the true event time in group k follows an exponential distribution with survival function $S_k(t; \lambda_k) = \exp(-\lambda_k t)$. The parameter λ_k here can be interpreted as the event rate in a prespecified time unit such as monthly or annual hazard rate. Recall that the τ-quantile residual lifetime at a given time t_0 under the exponential distribution is given by $-\log(1 - \tau)/\lambda_k$, which does not depend on t_0. Let us assume that the event times T_k are independent of the common censoring times C, which has the survival function $G(t; \eta) = \exp(-\eta t)$. By extending the results in Example 3.2 to the general τ-quantile case, the variance of the τ-quantile residual life estimator for group k is given by

$$V_k = \frac{\{\log(1-\tau)\}^2}{-n_k\lambda_k^2 \int_0^\infty G(v;\eta)dS_k(v;\lambda_k)} = \frac{\{\log(1-\tau)\}^2}{n_k\lambda_k^2\left(\frac{\lambda_k}{\lambda_k+\eta}\right)}, \tag{6.3}$$

where n_k is the sample size for group k. Here note that

$$\Pr(T_k \leq C) = -\int_0^\infty G(v;\eta)dS_k(v;\lambda_k) = \lambda_k/(\lambda_k+\eta)$$

is the *total* probability of occurrence of events in group k.

When the preliminary data are available from a pilot study, the variance in denominator of the test statistic $W_\alpha(\tau)$ can be estimated from the pooled sample under the null hypothesis. Specifically for the exponential case being considered here, the parameter λ_k ($k = 1,2$) can be replaced by its pooled estimate $\hat{\lambda}_{(pooled)} = d/\sum_{k=1}^2\sum_{i=1}^n x_{ki}$, where d is the total number of events across two groups and x_{ki} is the follow-up time for the ith subject in group k, either event or censored. When there are no preliminary data available, however, the simple average of λ_1 and λ_2 might be reasonable to be assumed because the total sample size n would be split evenly between two groups in a well-executed randomized study.

Now by replacing λ_k by $\lambda_0 = (\lambda_1 + \lambda_2)/2$ in (6.3), Eq. (6.2) can be rewritten as

$$z_{1-\frac{\alpha}{2}} - \frac{\Delta_1}{\sqrt{\left(\frac{1}{n_1}+\frac{1}{n_2}\right)\frac{\{\log(1-\tau)\}^2}{\lambda_0^2\left(\frac{\lambda_0}{\lambda_0+\eta}\right)}}} = z_\beta.$$

Assuming that $n_1 \approx n_2$, we have

$$n_1\left(\frac{\lambda_0}{\lambda_0+\eta}\right) \approx 2\left(\frac{z_{1-\frac{\alpha}{2}} - z_\beta}{\Delta_1}\right)^2\left\{\frac{\log(1-\tau)}{\lambda_0}\right\}^2.$$

Here $\lambda_0/(\lambda_0+\eta) = \Pr(T \leq C|H_0)$ is the pooled probability of occurrence of events in both groups combined under the null hypothesis. Therefore the total required number of events for both groups is given by

$$d = n\left(\frac{\lambda_0}{\lambda_0+\eta}\right) \approx 4\left(\frac{z_{1-\frac{\alpha}{2}} - z_\beta}{\Delta_1}\right)^2\left\{\frac{\log(1-\tau)}{\lambda_0}\right\}^2, \tag{6.4}$$

which also gives the total number of subjects as

$$n \approx 4 \left(\frac{z_{1-\frac{\alpha}{2}} - z_\beta}{\Delta_1} \right)^2 \left\{ \frac{\log(1 - \tau)}{\lambda_0} \right\}^2 \left(1 + \frac{\eta}{\lambda_0} \right). \qquad (6.5)$$

This implies that when the censoring rate in a specific time unit η is 0, the required number of subjects would be identical to the number of events. However, as the censoring rate becomes greater than 0, the number of subjects will be always larger than the number of events.

In fact, the sample size formula (6.4) can be re-expressed in terms of the hazard ratio. Since $\Delta_1 = -\log(1 - \tau)(1/\lambda_1 - 1/\lambda_2)$ and $\lambda_0 = (\lambda_1 + \lambda_2)/2$, denoting the hazard ratio by $\theta = \lambda_2/\lambda_1$ the formula (6.4) reduces to

$$d = 4 \left\{ \frac{z_{1-\frac{\alpha}{2}} - z_\beta}{\left(\frac{\theta^2 - 1}{2\theta} \right)} \right\}^2, \qquad (6.6)$$

which resembles the sample size formula based on the log-rank test,

$$d_{LR} = 4 \left\{ \frac{z_{1-\frac{\alpha}{2}} - z_\beta}{\log(\theta)} \right\}^2. \qquad (6.7)$$

One can show that the formula (6.6) always gives a smaller sample size, expectedly, than the formula (6.7) does, because $|(\theta^2 - 1)/(2\theta)| \geq \log(\theta)$ when $0 < \theta < 2$. This can be easily seen by using Taylor expansion of $\log(x)$ around $x = 1$ that gives $\log(x) \approx x - 1 - (1/2)(x - 1)^2 + \ldots$. By using the Taylor series approximation, the difference of the two functions can be written as

$$\frac{x^2 - 1}{2x} - \log(x) \approx \frac{(x - 1)^3}{2x}, \qquad 0 < x \leq 2,$$

which implies that $(x^2 - 1)/(2x) > \log(x)$ if $x > 1$ and $(x^2 - 1)/(2x) < \log(x)$ if $x < 1$.

The formula (6.4) also has an additional advantage in that it can be used to design a study to detect a quantile residual life difference directly. Specifically, again because

$$\Delta_1 = -\log(1 - \tau)(1/\lambda_1 - 1/\lambda_2)$$

$$= -\log(1 - \tau) \left(\frac{\theta - 1}{\theta \lambda_1} \right),$$

once the hazard rate for the control group (λ_1) and the quantile residual life to be detected (Δ_1) are specified, the hazard ratio θ, and hence λ_2, is accordingly determined, but it would not be of direct interest.

Example 6.1 (Comparison with Log-rank Test): In this example, we compare the proposed method based on a difference in the median residual lifetimes $(\tau = 1/2)$ and one based on the commonly used log-rank test statistic that tests for the logarithm of the hazard ratio. Suppose that the hazard rate for the control group is $\lambda_1 = 0.05$ and we want to detect 30% reduction in the hazard rate in the experimental group, i.e. $\lambda_2 = 0.035$, with 80% power with a two-sided 5% type I error probability. In this setting, the median residual lifetimes at any given time point for the control and experimental group would be constant as $\log(2)/0.05 = 13.9$ and $\log(2)/0.035 = 19.8$, respectively. Therefore we want to determine the required number of events to detect $\Delta_1 = 6$-year difference in the median residual lifetimes between the two groups, possibly, due to an intervention such as treatment by a new drug. With the pooled hazard rate $\lambda_0 = 0.0425$, the formula (6.4) gives the desired number of events of $d = 369$. Since $\theta = 0.67$ in our example, the required number of events based on the log-rank test statistic from (6.7) is $d_{LR} = 379$. One can see that both methods provide similar results, as expected, but the approach based on the two-sample test comparing the median residual lifetimes seems a little more efficient.

Given the accrual and event rates, there are two ways to reach the required number of events: (1) accrue the patients for a longer time period, which would increase the total number of subjects, and hence more events will occur faster and (2) fix the accrual period and hence the total number of subjects, but follow the accrued patients up for a longer time period until the required number of events is reached. Thus, once the total required number of events and the patient accrual rate is determined, based on the hypothesized event rate in each group, the duration of the study, including both accrual and follow-up periods, and the total number of subjects required can also be projected simultaneously. In a phase III clinical trial on breast cancer, for example, it would be reasonable to have a 2- to 3-years of the accrual period and follow the patients for another 2–3 years until the final analysis, the entire study period being 5–6 years.

6.2 Sample Size Calculation Under Competing Risks

In this section, we consider sample size calculation for a study to compare two quantile residual lifetimes under competing risks. We will be assuming that there are two types of competing events, type 1 and type 2, and interested in determining the number of events of type 1 events. For simplification, we will follow the cause-specific parametrization approach discussed in Sect. 4.3.1 and assume exponential distributions for both event type distributions, but different event rates, i.e. λ_1 for type 1 and λ_2 for type 2. We will also assume that the independent censoring distribution follows an exponential distribution with the rate parameter η.

Let us define $q_{1k} = \theta_{1,t_0}^{(k)}(\tau; \boldsymbol{\psi}^{(k)})$ to be the τ-quantile from a residual life distribution for group k ($k = 1, 2$) at time t_0, defined in (4.19) under the cause-specific exponential formulation, and $V_{1k} = \mathrm{Var}(\hat{q}_{1k})$, where $\hat{q}_{1k} = \theta_{1,t_0}^{(k)}(\tau; \widehat{\boldsymbol{\psi}}^{(k)})$. Similarly as in the previous section, under the null hypothesis $H_0 : \Delta = q_{11} - q_{12} = 0$, the two-sample statistic $W_{1,t_0}(\tau) = (\hat{q}_{11} - \hat{q}_{12})/\sqrt{V_{11} + V_{12}}$ can be used to derive the sample size formula under the asymptotic normality assumption.

Suppose that we want to detect a τ-quantile difference $\Delta = \Delta_{11} = q_{11} - q_{12}$ between two residual life distributions of type 1 events under competing risks by using a two-sided test with type I error probability of α. Following the similar arguments as in the previous section, Eq. (6.2) can be modified to

$$z_{1-\frac{\alpha}{2}} - \frac{\Delta_{11}}{\sqrt{V_{11} + V_{12}}} = z_\beta. \tag{6.8}$$

From Sect. 4.3.1, the variance of $\hat{q}_{1k}$ is given by

$$
V_{1k} = \left(\frac{\lambda_{1k}^2}{\sum_{i=1}^{n_1} \delta_{1i}^{(k)}}\right) \left\{\frac{\log\left(1 - \tau e^{-\lambda_{2k}t_0}\right)}{\lambda_{1k}^2}\right\}^2
$$
$$
+ \left(\frac{\lambda_{2k}^2}{\sum_{i=1}^{n_2} \delta_{2i}^{(k)}}\right) \left\{\frac{\tau t_0 e^{-\lambda_{2k}t_0}}{\lambda_{1k}(1 - \tau e^{-\lambda_{2k}t_0})}\right\}^2, \tag{6.9}
$$

where $\delta_{ji}^{(k)} = I(T_i^{(k)} < C, \epsilon = j)$ is the type j event indicator for the ith subject in group k.

We need to first find the expectation of $\delta_{ji}^{(k)}$ in (6.9), i.e. for two competing event times $T_{1i}^{(k)}$ and $T_{2i}^{(k)}$ and the common censoring time C_i,

$$
\begin{aligned}
E(\delta_{1i}) &= E[I(T_{1i}^{(k)} < T_{2i}^{(k)} \text{ and } T_{1i}^{(k)} < C_i)] \\
&= \Pr(T_{1i}^{(k)} < T_{2i}^{(k)} \text{ and } T_{1i}^{(k)} < C_i) \\
&= E[\Pr(T_{1i}^{(k)} < T_{2i}^{(k)} \text{ and } T_{1i}^{(k)} < C_i | T_{1i}^{(k)} = t)] \\
&= E\left[\frac{\Pr(T_{2i}^{(k)} > t, C_i > t, T_{1i}^{(k)} = t)}{\Pr(T_{1i}^{(k)} = t)}\right]
\end{aligned} \tag{6.10}
$$

Assuming that the type 1 and type 2 event times and the censoring time are independent, the expectation in (6.10) can be written as

$$
E\left[\frac{\Pr(T_{2i}^{(k)} > t, T_{1i}^{(k)} = t)\Pr(C_i > t)}{\Pr(T_{1i}^{(k)} = t)}\right].
$$

Under the cause-specific parameterization, from Sect. 4.3.1, since $\Pr(T_{2i}^{(k)} > t, T_{1i}^{(k)} = t)$ is equivalent to $\Pr(\min(T_{1i}^{(k)}, T_{2i}^{(k)}) = t, j = 1) = \Pr(\min(T_{1i}^{(k)}, T_{2i}^{(k)}) \geq t)h_1^{(k)}(t) = S^{(k)}(t-)h_1^{(k)}(t) = f_1^{(k)}(t) = \Pr(T_{1i}^{(k)} = t)$, we finally have

$$
E(\delta_{1i}^{(k)}) = E\left[\Pr(C_i > t)\right] = -\int_0^\infty G(v)dS_1^{(k)}(v), \tag{6.11}
$$

where $G(v)$ is the survival function of the censoring distribution and $S_1^{(k)}(v)$ is the cause-specific survival function for type 1 events in group k. Assuming that the cause-specific distribution for type 1 events follows an exponential distribution with the rate parameter λ_{1k} and the censoring distribution follows an exponential distribution with the rate parameter η, the expectation (6.11) reduces to

$$E(\delta_{1i}^{(k)}) = \int_0^\infty \lambda_{1k} e^{-(\lambda_{1k}+\eta)v} dv = \frac{\lambda_{1k}}{\lambda_{1k}+\eta}. \qquad (6.12)$$

By defining the pooled event rates as $\lambda_{10} = (\lambda_{11} + \lambda_{12})/2$ and $\lambda_{20} = (\lambda_{21} + \lambda_{22})/2$ under the null hypothesis, and by using (6.9), $V_{11} + V_{12}$ can be simplified to

$$2\left[\left(\frac{\lambda_{10}^2}{n_1\pi_1}\right) \left\{ \frac{\log\left(1 - \tau e^{-\lambda_{20}t_0}\right)}{\lambda_{10}^2} \right\}^2 \right.$$
$$\left. + \left(\frac{\lambda_{20}^2}{n_2\pi_2}\right) \left\{ \frac{\tau t_0 e^{-\lambda_{20}t_0}}{\lambda_{10}(1 - \tau e^{-\lambda_{20}t_0})} \right\}^2 \right],$$

where $\pi_1 = \lambda_{10}/(\lambda_{10} + \eta)$ and $\pi_2 = \lambda_{20}/(\lambda_{20} + \eta)$ are the total probabilities of type 1 and type 2 events under the null hypothesis. Further assuming that $n_2 = n_1 = n/2$ and $\pi_2 = \phi\pi_1$, Eq. (6.8) gives

$$2\left[\left(\frac{\lambda_{10}^2}{n_1\pi_1}\right) \left\{ \frac{\log\left(1 - \tau e^{-\lambda_{20}t_0}\right)}{\lambda_{10}^2} \right\}^2 \right.$$
$$\left. + \left(\frac{\lambda_{20}^2}{n_1\phi\pi_1}\right) \left\{ \frac{\tau t_0 e^{-\lambda_{20}t_0}}{\lambda_{10}(1 - \tau e^{-\lambda_{20}t_0})} \right\}^2 \right]$$
$$= \left(\frac{\Delta_{11}}{z_{1-\alpha/2} - z_\beta}\right)^2,$$

which gives the required number of type 1 events, d_1, as

$$d_1 = n\pi_1 = 4\left(\frac{z_{1-\alpha/2} - z_\beta}{\Delta_{11}}\right)^2 \left[\left\{ \frac{\log\left(1 - \tau e^{-\lambda_{20}t_0}\right)}{\lambda_{10}} \right\}^2 \right.$$
$$\left. + \left(\frac{1}{\phi}\right) \left\{ \frac{\tau \lambda_{20} t_0 e^{-\lambda_{20}t_0}}{\lambda_{10}(1 - \tau e^{-\lambda_{20}t_0})} \right\}^2 \right]. \qquad (6.13)$$

One can notice that this formula reduces to (6.4) with λ_0 replaced by λ_{10}, the pooled cause-specific hazard rate for type 1 events, when $t_0 = 0$, which would be of most interest in practice, even though the formula (6.13) provides a panoramic view about how the sample size would be changed if the study is designed at a different time point.

When $t_0 = 0$, the sample size formula (6.13) reduces to

$$d_1 = 4 \left(\frac{z_{1-\alpha/2} - z_\beta}{\Delta_{11}} \right)^2 \left\{ \frac{\log(1 - \tau)}{\lambda_{10}} \right\}^2,$$

which can be re-expressed similarly as before in terms of the cause-specific hazard ratio of type 1 events, $\theta_1 = \lambda_{12}/\lambda_{11}$ as

$$d_1 = 4 \left\{ \frac{z_{1-\frac{\alpha}{2}} - z_\beta}{\left(\frac{\theta_1^2 - 1}{2\theta_1} \right)} \right\}^2, \tag{6.14}$$

because

$$\Delta_{11} = -\log(1 - \tau) \left(\frac{1}{\lambda_{11}} - \frac{1}{\lambda_{12}} \right) = -\log(1 - \tau) \left(\frac{\theta_1 - 1}{\theta_1 \lambda_{11}} \right), \tag{6.15}$$

and $\lambda_{10} = (\lambda_{11} + \lambda_{12})/2$. Again once the cause-specific hazard rate for type 1 events in the control group (λ_{11}) and the difference in τ-quantile failure times of the distribution of type 1 events between two groups to be detected (Δ_{11}) are specified, the cause-specific hazard ratio (θ_1) and hence the cause-specific hazard rate of type 1 events for the experimental group (λ_{12}) are implicitly determined in Eq. (6.15). Also the formula (6.14) would provide a smaller sample size than one based on the log-rank test statistic under competing risks.

Appendix: R Codes

In this chapter, we include the R codes that were used in the examples throughout the book.

A.1 Example 3.3 in Sect. 3.5.1

```
## Functions to extract Kaplan-Meier estimates
## corresponding to survival probabilities x

fct.q1.t0<-function(x){km.1$time[km.1$surv <= x][1]}

library(survival)
library(base)

# Setting up the parameter values
lambda<-0.09
kappa<-2

# Setting up the number of observations
n.obs<-10

# Fixed time point for residual life distribution
t0<-2.0

# Data generation (a=1.5 and b=10 for the censoring
# distribution)
set.seed(1234)
```

J.-H. Jeong, *Statistical Inference on Residual Life*,
Statistics for Biology and Health, DOI 10.1007/978-1-4939-0005-3,
© Springer Science+Business Media New York 2014

```
u.1<-runif(n.obs)
time<-(-(1/lambda)*log(1-u.1))^(1/kappa)
cens<-runif(n.obs,1.5,10)
event<-c(rep(0,n.obs))
event[time <= cens]<-1
new.time<-apply(cbind(time,cens),1,min)
time.obs<-new.time

data.tmp<-data.frame(cbind(time.obs,event))

my.data<-round(data.tmp[order(data.tmp[,1]),],3)

# Kaplan-Meier estimates
km.1<-survfit(Surv(time.obs,event)~1,data=my.data)
# Kaplan-Meier estimate at t0=2
surv.t0<-min(km.1$surv[km.1$time <= t0])
# Estimate of the quantile residual life at t0=2
q1.t0<-fct.q1.t0(surv.t0/2)-t0

surv.t0/2
#[1] 0.35
fct.q1.t0(surv.t0/2)
#[1] 3.293963
q1.t0
#[1] 1.293963

# Creating Figure 3.5
plot(km.1,xlab="Time",ylab="Probability of Event-free")

# Calculation of 95% confidence interval from one-sample
# test statistic
unique.1<-data.frame(cbind(km.1$time,km.1$n.event,
  km.1$n.risk,km.1$surv))
names(unique.1)<-c("time","dN","y","k-m")

unique.1$indi.0.t0<-rep(0,length(unique.1[,1]))
unique.1$indi.0.t0[unique.1$time >= 0 & unique.1$time
  <= t0]<-1

unique.1$indi.0.q1.t0<-rep(0,length(unique.1[,1]))
```

```
unique.1$indi.0.q1.t0[unique.1$time >= 0 & unique.1$time
    <= t0+q1.t0]<-1

unique.1$indi.t0.q1.t0<-rep(0,length(unique.1[,1]))
unique.1$indi.t0.q1.t0[unique.1$time >= t0 & unique.1$time
    <= t0+q1.t0]<-1

names(unique.1)<-c("time","dN","y","k-m","indi.0.t0",
"indi.0.q1.t0", "indi.t0.q1.t0")

term.11<-(unique.1$indi.0.q1.t0*unique.1$dN)/unique.1$y
term.12<-cumsum((unique.1$indi.0.q1.t0*unique.1$dN)
      /unique.1$y^2)
epsilon.i1<--min(km.1$surv[km.1$time <= t0+q1.t0])
     *(term.11-term.12)

term.21<-(unique.1$indi.0.t0*unique.1$dN)/unique.1$y
term.22<-cumsum((unique.1$indi.0.t0*unique.1$dN)
                /unique.1$y^2)
epsilon.i2<-(1/2)*surv.t0*(term.21-term.22)

epsilon.i<-epsilon.i1+epsilon.i2

var.1<-sum(epsilon.i^2)
var.1
#[1] 0.01022456

time.max.0<-max(time.obs)-t0
support.points.0<-seq(0,time.max.0,0.01)
disp.0<-apply(as.matrix(support.points.0),1,function(x)
{(summary(km.1,times=t0+x)$surv-(1/2)*surv.t0)^2/var.1})

covered.q0<-support.points.0[disp.0 < qchisq(0.95,1)]
# 95% confidence interval when n.obs=10
c(min(covered.q0),max(covered.q0)) # 95% confidence
                                   # interval
c(min(covered.q0),max(covered.q0))
#[1] 1.24 1.37


# Calculating the true quantile residual life at t0=2
```

```
true.q<-lambda^(-1/kappa)*(log(2)+lambda*t0^kappa)^
  (1/kappa)-t0
true.q
#[1] 1.420765

## Recalculation of 95% confidence interval when n.obs=100
c(min(covered.q0),max(covered.q0))
#[1] 0.81 1.62
```

A.2   Example 3.4 in Sect. 3.5.2

```
## Functions to extract Kaplan-Meier estimates
## corresponding to survival probabilities x

fct.q1.t0<-function(x){km.1$time[km.1$surv <= x][1]}
fct.q2.t0<-function(x){km.2$time[km.2$surv <= x][1]}

library(survival)
library(base)

# Setting up the parameter values
lambda<-0.09
kappa<-2

# Setting up the number of observations
n.obs<-100

# Fixing a time point for the residual life distribution
t0<-2

# Data generation (an identical distribution for both
# groups)
set.seed(1234)
u.0<-runif(n.obs)
u.1<-runif(n.obs)
time.0<-(-(1/lambda)*log(1-u.1))^(1/kappa)
time.1<-(-(1/lambda)*log(1-u.1))^(1/kappa)
time<-c(time.0,time.1)
```

```
cens<-runif(2*n.obs,1.5,10)
event<-c(rep(0,2*n.obs))
event[time <= cens]<-1
new.time<-apply(cbind(time,cens),1,min)
group<-c(rep(0,n.obs),rep(1,n.obs))
time.obs<-new.time

data.tmp<-data.frame(cbind(time.obs,group,event))

data.tmp.new<-round(data.tmp[order(data.tmp[,1]),],3)

## Evaluating the two-sample statistic under the null
## hypothesis and estimating 95% confidence intervals
## by converting it

# Group 1
my.data<-data.tmp.new[data.tmp.new$group==0,]
km.1<-survfit(Surv(time.obs,event)~1,data=my.data)
surv.t0<-min(km.1$surv[km.1$time <= t0])
q1.t0<-fct.q1.t0(surv.t0/2)-t0

surv.t0/2
fct.q1.t0(surv.t0/2)
q1.t0

#> surv.t0/2
#[1] 0.3735127
#> fct.q1.t0(surv.t0/2)
#[1] 3.332
#> q1.t0
#[1] 1.332

unique.1<-data.frame(cbind(km.1$time,km.1$n.event,km.1$n.
                     risk,km.1$surv))
names(unique.1)<-c("time","dN","y","k-m")

unique.1$indi.0.t0<-rep(0,length(unique.1[,1]))
unique.1$indi.0.t0[unique.1$time >= 0 & unique.1$time
                   <= t0]<-1
```

```
unique.1$indi.0.q1.t0<-rep(0,length(unique.1[,1]))
unique.1$indi.0.q1.t0[unique.1$time >= 0 & unique.1$time
                <= t0+q1.t0]<-1

names(unique.1)<-c("time","dN","y","k-m","indi.0.t0",
                "indi.0.q1.t0")

term.11<-(unique.1$indi.0.q1.t0*unique.1$dN)/unique.1$y
term.12<-cumsum((unique.1$indi.0.q1.t0*unique.1$dN)
                /unique.1$y^2)
epsilon.i1<--min(km.1$surv[km.1$time <= t0+q1.t0])*
                (term.11-term.12)

term.21<-(unique.1$indi.0.t0*unique.1$dN)/unique.1$y
term.22<-cumsum((unique.1$indi.0.t0*unique.1$dN)
                /unique.1$y^2)
epsilon.i2<-(1/2)*surv.t0*(term.21-term.22)

epsilon.i<-epsilon.i1+epsilon.i2

var.1<-sum(epsilon.i^2)

## Group 2
my.data<-data.tmp.new[data.tmp.new$group==1,]
km.2<-survfit(Surv(time.obs,event)~1,data=my.data)
surv.t0<-min(km.2$surv[km.2$time <= t0])
q2.t0<-fct.q2.t0(surv.t0/2)-t0

surv.t0/2
fct.q2.t0(surv.t0/2)
q2.t0

#> surv.t0/2
#[1] 0.3726659
#> fct.q2.t0(surv.t0/2)
#[1] 3.357
#> q2.t0
#[1] 1.357
```

```
unique.1<-data.frame(cbind(km.2$time,km.2$n.event,
                     km.2$n.risk,km.2$surv))
names(unique.1)<-c("time","dN","y","k-m")

unique.1$indi.0.t0<-rep(0,length(unique.1[,1]))
unique.1$indi.0.t0[unique.1$time >= 0 & unique.1$time
                   <= t0]<-1

unique.1$indi.0.q2.t0<-rep(0,length(unique.1[,1]))
unique.1$indi.0.q2.t0[unique.1$time >= 0 & unique.1$time
                      <= t0+q2.t0]<-1

names(unique.1)<-c("time","dN","y","k-m","indi.0.t0",
                   "indi.0.q2.t0")

term.11<-(unique.1$indi.0.q2.t0*unique.1$dN)/unique.1$y
term.12<-cumsum((unique.1$indi.0.q2.t0*unique.1$dN)
               /unique.1$y^2)
epsilon.i1<--min(km.2$surv[km.2$time <= t0+q2.t0])
                *(term.11-term.12)

term.21<-(unique.1$indi.0.t0*unique.1$dN)/unique.1$y
term.22<-cumsum((unique.1$indi.0.t0*unique.1$dN)
               /unique.1$y^2)
epsilon.i2<-(1/2)*surv.t0*(term.21-term.22)

epsilon.i<-epsilon.i1+epsilon.i2

var.2<-sum(epsilon.i^2)

eta<-seq(0,10,0.01)
time.max<-max(time.obs)
support.points<-seq(0,time.max,0.01)
term.1<-(summary(km.1,times=support.points+t0)$surv
-0.5*summary(km.1,times=t0)$surv)^2/var.1

support.matrix.group2<-apply(as.matrix(eta),1,
                       function(x){x*support.points})
min.dispersion.eta<-apply(support.matrix.group2,2,
                       function(x){
```

```
term.2<-(summary(km.2,times=x+t0)$surv-0.5*summary
             (km.2,times=t0)$surv)^2/var.2;
support.limit<-min(length(term.1),length(term.2))
 test.stat<-cbind(support.points[1:support.limit],
                     term.1[1:support.limit]
+term.2[1:support.limit]);
 min.rows<-as.numeric(test.stat[test.stat[,2]==
                     min(test.stat[,2]),])
min.rows[length(min.rows)]
})


covered.q0<-support.points[min.dispersion.eta <=
                     qchisq(0.95,1)]
# 95% confidence interval for the ratio of two median
# residual lifetimes
c(min(covered.q0),max(covered.q0))
#[1] 0.64 1.62


# Evaluated two sample statistic under the null hypothesis
min.dispersion.eta[eta==1]
#[1] 0.2154452


## Creating Figure 3.6
plot(eta[1:500],min.dispersion.eta[1:500],type="l",lty=1,
xlab="Ratio of two medians",ylab="Two-sample Statistic")
abline(h=qchisq(0.95,1),lty=2)
```

A.3   Example 3.11 in Sect. 3.6.3

```
MMRRegEst <- function(x, U, delta, tzero, LS=TRUE,
             tau=0.5) {
# This R function computes the residual median/mean case
# weighted regression estimator for randomly right
# censored data. It can compute the least squares
# estimator or quantile regression estimator. In the
# later case, it calls a function in the quantreg()
# package.
# Input:
```

```
# x: is a matrix of N rows (covariates). Intercept,
# if needed, has to be added explicitly.
# U: is the observed (censored) responses, No log
# transformation.
#         The code will later apply a log transformation
# after getting the residual times.
# delta: is a vector of length N. delta =1 means (U) is
#            not censored. delta = 0 means U is
#            right censored, i.e. the true response is
#            larger than U.
# tzero:  the residual life after this time. Same as t_0
# in the text.
# LS: is logical. indicates if this is a least square
#       regression or quantile regression.
# tau: if LS=TRUE then this is ignored, otherwise tau is
# used in rqfit.
#
# Output:
# the estimates of regression parameters, \hat beta.

n <- length(U)
x <- as.matrix(x)
xdim <- dim(x)
if ( xdim[1] != n ) stop("check dim of x")
if ( length(delta) != n ) stop("check length of delta")
if(any((delta!=0)&(delta!=1)))
    stop("delta must be 0(right-censored) or
         1(uncensored)")

temp <- WKM(x=U, d=delta, zc=1:n)
KMweight <- temp$jump
norder <- order(U, -delta)
ZZ <- U[norder]
residualAfter <- as.numeric( ZZ > tzero )
KMweight <- KMweight*residualAfter

### the zero weights should be removed
Wplace <- which(KMweight > 0)
if( length(Wplace) <= 3) stop("too few uncensored Y that
        exceed tzero")
```

```
KMweight <- KMweight[Wplace]
ZZ <- ZZ[Wplace] - tzero
ZZ <- log(ZZ)   #### or some other transformation,
          log10(ZZ) etc
XX <- as.matrix(x[norder,])
xmat <- as.matrix(XX[Wplace,])
if(LS) estim <- coef(lm.wfit(x=xmat, y=ZZ, w=KMweight))
if(!LS) estim <- coef(rq.wfit(x=xmat, y=ZZ,
                        weights=KMweight, tau=tau))
return(estim)
}


## Data Generaton ##

total.size<-20

time.temp<-rep(0,total.size)
x1<-rep(0,total.size) # covariate 1
rho<-rep(0,total.size)
u<-rep(0,total.size)
cens<-rep(0,total.size)
death<-rep(0,total.size)
new.time<-rep(0,total.size)

intercept<-1.609438 # true intercept value, so that
      exp(1.609438)=5
beta1<-0 # true beta_1 value
kappa<-2.0
cens.para<-52

t.fixed<-0     # A time point where the median residual
                # lifetime is estimated.

set.seed(3224)

for (i in 1:total.size){
x1[i]<-floor(round(runif(1,0,1))) # Covariate (binary)
rho[i]<-log(2)*(exp(intercept+beta1*x1[i]))^(-kappa)
u[i]<-runif(1,0,1)
time.temp[i]<-(-log(1-u[i])/rho[i])^(1/kappa)
```

```
cens[i]<-runif(1,0, cens.para)
death[i]<-ifelse(time.temp[i] <= cens[i],1,0)
new.time[i]<-min(time.temp[i],cens[i])
}
temp.dat<-data.frame(cbind(time.temp,x1,cens,death,
                          new.time))
temp<-round(temp.dat[order(temp.dat$new.time),],3)

## Estimation ##

library(emplik)
para<-MMRRegEst(x=cbind(1,temp$x1),U=temp$new.time,
delta=temp$death, LS=F, tau=0.5, tzero=t.fixed)
para
#[1]  1.6420987 -0.4221541

# When sample size=500
para
#[1]   1.60341984 -0.01357258

## Calculating the variance-covariance matrix of
## score functions for the global test

library(survival)
time.obs<-new.time
z.original<-cbind(rep(1,length(x1)),x1)
beta.hat<-para
reg.line.hat<-exp(z.original%*%beta.hat) # exp(beta.hat*z)
t.beta.z<-t.fixed+reg.line.hat[order(reg.line.hat)]
                                # t+exp(beta.hat*z)
time<-time.obs[order(reg.line.hat)]
death.new<-death[order(reg.line.hat)]
z<-z.original[order(reg.line.hat),]
km.cens.new<-survfit(Surv(time,1-death.new)~1)
indi.1.new<-as.numeric(time >= t.beta.z)
indi.2.new<-as.numeric(time >= t.fixed)
is.in.range<-t.beta.z >= min(time) & t.beta.z <= max(time)
km.cens.1.new<-
  ifelse(is.in.range,summary(km.cens.new,time=
              c(t.beta.z[is.in.range]))$surv,
```

```
min(summary(km.cens.new)$surv))
km.cens.1.new[t.beta.z < min(time)]<-1
 km.cens.1.new[km.cens.1.new==0]<-sort(summary
               (km.cens.new)$surv)[2]
km.cens.2.new<-ifelse(t.fixed <=
  max(time),summary(km.cens.new,time=c(t.fixed))$surv,
min(summary(km.cens.new)$surv))
 term1<-z*(indi.1.new/km.cens.1.new-indi.2.new
             /(2*km.cens.2.new))
term22<-matrix(rep(0,total.size^2),ncol=total.size)
term32<-matrix(rep(0,total.size^2),ncol=total.size)
sum.risk<-apply(as.matrix(time),1,function(x)
             {sum(x <= time)})
 term21<-t(apply(as.matrix(time),1,function(x)
           {(1-death.new[time==x])*
(x <= t.beta.z)/sum(x <= time)}))
 term31<-t(apply(as.matrix(time),1,function(x)
           {(1-death.new[time==x])*
(x <= rep(t.fixed,total.size))/sum(x <= time)}))
min.temp22<-apply(as.matrix(time),1,function(x)
 {apply(matrix(c(rep(x,length(time)),t.beta.z),
        ncol=2),1,min)})
term22<-apply(as.matrix(min.temp22),1,function(x)
             {apply((1-
death.new)*(apply(as.matrix(x),1,function(y){time <= y})
             /sum.risk^2),2,sum)})
min.temp32<-apply(as.matrix(time),1,function(x)
 {apply(matrix(c(rep(x,length(time)),rep(t.fixed,
        length(time))),ncol=2),1,min)})
term32<-apply(as.matrix(min.temp32),1,function(x)
          {apply((1-
death.new)*(apply(as.matrix(x),1,function(y){time <= y})
        /sum.risk^2),2,sum)})
temp.z1<-(indi.1.new/km.cens.1.new)*z
temp.term2<-term21-term22
term2<-temp.term2%*%temp.z1
temp.z2<-(indi.2.new/(2*total.size*km.cens.2.new))*z
temp.term3<-term31-term32
term3<-temp.term3%*%temp.z2
tau<-term1+term2-term3
```

```
variance<-(1/total.size)*t(tau)%*%tau

variance
#                      x1
#   0.2743142 0.1371484
#x1 0.1371484 0.1507630

## Calculating the global test statistic##

para.null<-c(0,0)
reg.line<-exp(z.original%*%para.null)  #exp(beta_hat*z)
time<-time.obs[order(reg.line)]
death.new<-death[order(reg.line)]
z<-z.original[order(reg.line),]
t.beta.z<-t.fixed+reg.line[order(reg.line)]
                                # t+exp(beta*z)
indi.1<-as.numeric(time >= t.beta.z)
indi.2<-as.numeric(time >= t.fixed)
km.cens<-survfit(Surv(time,1-death.new)~1)
is.in.range<-t.beta.z >= min(time) & t.beta.z <= max(time)
km.cens.1<-ifelse(is.in.range,summary(km.cens,
  time=c(t.beta.z[is.in.range]))$surv,min(summary(km.cens)
             $surv))
km.cens.1[t.beta.z < min(time)]<-1
km.cens.1[km.cens.1==0]<-sort(summary(km.cens)$surv)[2]
km.cens.2<-ifelse(t.fixed <= max(time),summary(km.cens,
  time=c(t.fixed))$surv,min(summary(km.cens)$surv))
global.stat<-((total.size)^(-1))*t(apply((indi.1/km.cens.
            1-indi.2/(2*km.cens.2))*z,2,sum))%*%
            solve(variance)%*%
apply((indi.1/km.cens.1-indi.2/(2*km.cens.2))*z,2,sum)

global.stat
#          [,1]
#[1,] 12.27347

qchisq(0.95,2)
#[1] 5.991465

## Calculating the minimum dispersion statistic for
```

```r
## testing the null hypothetsis for beta_2=0 (local test)

s.var<-function(b1){
reg.line<-exp(z.original%*%c(b1,b2))  #exp(beta*z)
time<-time.obs[order(reg.line)]
death.new<-death[order(reg.line)]
z<-z.original[order(reg.line),]
t.beta.z<-t.fixed+reg.line[order(reg.line)]
                                # t+exp(beta*z)
indi.1<-as.numeric(time >= t.beta.z)
indi.2<-as.numeric(time >= t.fixed)
km.cens<-survfit(Surv(time,1-death.new)~1)
is.in.range<-t.beta.z >= min(time) & t.beta.z <= max(time)
km.cens.1<-ifelse(is.in.range,summary(km.cens,
 time=c(t.beta.z[is.in.range]))$surv,min(summary
             (km.cens)$surv))
km.cens.1[t.beta.z < min(time)]<-1
km.cens.1[km.cens.1==0]<-sort(summary(km.cens)$surv)[2]
km.cens.2<-ifelse(t.fixed <= max(time),
 summary(km.cens,time=c(t.fixed))$surv,min(summary
             (km.cens)$surv))
((total.size)^(-1))*t(apply((indi.1/km.cens.1-
indi.2/(2*km.cens.2))*z,2,sum))%*%solve(variance)%*%
apply((indi.1/km.cens.1-indi.2/(2*km.cens.2))*z,2,sum)
}


b2<-0
old.init<-5.0
range<-5


l.limit.x<-old.init-range
u.limit.x<-old.init+range
incre.x<-(u.limit.x-l.limit.x)/5
n.points.x<-(1/incre.x)*((u.limit.x-l.limit.x)+incre.x)
b1<-seq(l.limit.x,u.limit.x,incre.x)
score<-apply(as.matrix(b1),1,s.var)
min.score.old<-min(score)
if(length(b1[score==min.score.old])>1) new.init<-
b1[score==min.score.old][1] else new.init<-b1[score==min.
          score.old]
```

```
range<-0.75*range
l.limit.x<-new.init-range
u.limit.x<-new.init+range
incre.x<-(u.limit.x-l.limit.x)/5
n.points.x<-(1/incre.x)*((u.limit.x-l.limit.x)+incre.x)
b1<-seq(l.limit.x,u.limit.x,incre.x)
score<-apply(as.matrix(b1),1,s.var)
min.score.new<-min(score)

while (abs(min.score.new-min.score.old) > 0.001){
if(length(b1[score==min.score.new])>1) new.init<-
b1[score==min.score.new][1] else new.init<-
        b1[score==min.score.new]

range<-0.75*range

l.limit.x<-new.init-range
u.limit.x<-new.init+range
incre.x<-(u.limit.x-l.limit.x)/5
n.points.x<-(1/incre.x)*((u.limit.x-l.limit.x)+incre.x)
b1<-seq(l.limit.x,u.limit.x,incre.x)
score<-apply(as.matrix(b1),1,s.var)
min.score.old<-min.score.new
min.score.new<-min(score)
}

min.disp<-min.score.new
min.disp
#[1] 0.9491851

qchisq(0.95, 1)
#[1] 3.841459

## Generating Table 3.4

tbl.1<-data.frame(cbind(temp$new.time,temp$death,temp$x1))
names(tbl.1)<-c("Time","Event Indicator",
                "Group Indicator")
tbl.1
```

A.4   Example 4.3 in Sect. 4.3.1

```
## Functions to select a cuminc estimate (Gray) at a
## fixed time x when there are two trt groups and
## two types of events. First subscript is group
## (0=control;1=active) and second subscript is type of
## events (1=of  interest (F1); 2=other (F2))

cuminc.01<-function(x){
max(xx[[1]]$est[xx[[1]]$time <= x])
}
cuminc.02<-function(x){
max(xx[[2]]$est[xx[[2]]$time <= x])
}


## Functions to invert the cuminc estimates (Gray) when
## there are two trt groups and two types of events. First
## subscript is group (0=control;1=active) and second
## subscript is type of events (1=of interest (F1);
## 2=other (F2))

inv.cuminc.01<-function(x){
min(xx[[1]]$time[xx[[1]]$est >= x])
}
inv.cuminc.02<-function(x){
min(xx[[2]]$time[xx[[2]]$est >= x])
}


## Data Generation
generate.data<-function(n.obs,pi.1,lambda.1,kappa.1,
                        lambda.2,kappa.2,cens)
{
set.seed(3224)
binom.number<-rbinom(n.obs,1,pi.1)
u.1<-runif(as.numeric(table(binom.number)[1]),0,1)
u.2<-runif(as.numeric(table(binom.number)[2]),0,1)
time<-rep(NA,n.obs)
time[binom.number==0]<-(-(1/lambda.1)*log(1-u.1))
                       ^(1/kappa.1)
```

```
time[binom.number==1]<-(-(1/lambda.2)*log(1-u.2))
                        ^(1/kappa.2)
censored<-runif(n.obs,0,cens)
obs.time<-apply(cbind(time,censored),1,min)
event.i<-rep(NA,n.obs)
event.i[binom.number==0]<-1
event.i[binom.number==1]<-2
event.i[obs.time==censored]<-0
temp<-data.frame(cbind(obs.time,event.i))
}

temp<-generate.data(10,0.5,0.09,1.5,0.09,1.5,45)

names(temp)<-c("time","event")
my.data<-round(temp[order(temp$time),],3)

library(cmprsk)
xx <- cuminc(my.data$time,my.data$event)

## How to extract F_1(x) and F_2(x)
time.comb<-sort(my.data$time[my.data$event==1 |
          my.data$event==2])
F01.x<-apply(t(time.comb),2,cuminc.01)
F02.x<-apply(t(time.comb),2,cuminc.02)

km1.x<-(1-F01.x-F02.x) # This is equivalent to KM est.

p<-0.2
t0<-2

km.1.t0<-1-cuminc.01(t0)-cuminc.02(t0)
q1.t0<-inv.cuminc.01(cuminc.01(t0)+p*km.1.t0)-t0
#> q1.t0
#[1] 1.59

temp.surv.1<-survfit(Surv(my.data$time,my.data$event>0)~1)
temp.my<-my.data[!is.na(pmatch(my.data$time,
                temp.surv.1$time)),]
```

```
unique.1<-data.frame(cbind(temp.surv.1$time,
                    temp.surv.1$surv,
temp.surv.1$n.risk,temp.surv.1$n.event,temp.my$event))
names(unique.1)<-c("time","km.1.all","y","dN",
                    "event.type")

unique.1$indi.t0.q1.t0<-rep(0,length(unique.1[,1]))
unique.1$indi.t0.q1.t0[unique.1$time >= t0 &
unique.1$time <= t0+q1.t0]<-1

unique.1$indi.0.t0<-rep(0,length(unique.1[,1]))
unique.1$indi.0.t0[unique.1$time > 0 & unique.1$time
                                    <= t0]<-1

unique.1$indi.all.events<-rep(0,length(unique.1[,1]))
unique.1$indi.all.events[unique.1$event.type > 0]<-1

unique.1$indi.event.j<-rep(0,length(unique.1[,1]))
unique.1$indi.event.j[unique.1$event.type == 1]<-1

unique.1$dS.diff<-diff(c(0,unique.1$time))*
c(1,unique.1$km.1.all[1:c(length(unique.1$km.1.all)-1)])

term.1.1<-(unique.1$indi.t0.q1.t0*unique.1$km.1.all*
unique.1$indi.event.j)/unique.1$y
term.1.2<-cumsum((unique.1$indi.t0.q1.t0*
                    unique.1$km.1.all*
unique.1$indi.event.j)/unique.1$y^2)
term.1<-term.1.1-term.1.2

term.2.1<-unique.1$indi.t0.q1.t0*unique.1$dS.diff*
((unique.1$indi.event.j)/unique.1$y)
term.2.2<-unique.1$dS.diff*cumsum(unique.1$indi.t0.q1.t0*
(unique.1$indi.event.j)/unique.1$y^2)
term.2<-term.2.1-term.2.2

term.3.1<-p*km.1.t0*unique.1$indi.0.t0*
(unique.1$indi.all.events/unique.1$y)
term.3.2<-p*km.1.t0*cumsum(unique.1$indi.0.t0*
(unique.1$indi.all.events/unique.1$y^2))
```

```
term.3<-term.3.1-term.3.2

var.1<-sum((term.1-term.2-term.3)^2) # variance of u.1 in
          group 1
#> var.1
#[1] 0.008985795

time.max.0<-max(my.data$time)
support.points.0<-seq(0,time.max.0,0.01)
disp.0<-apply(as.matrix(support.points.0),1,function(x){
(cuminc.01(t0+x)-cuminc.01(t0)-p*km.1.t0)^2/var.1})

covered.q0<-support.points.0[disp.0 < qchisq(0.95,1)]

## 95% confidence interval for the 0.2-quantile of the
## residual life distribution of type 1 events

c(min(covered.q0),max(covered.q0))
#[1] 0.00 11.48 # Equivalent to (-infty, infty)

## 95% confidence interval when n=100

covered.q0<-support.points.0[disp.0 < qchisq(0.95,1)]
c(min(covered.q0),max(covered.q0)) # 95% ci
#[1] 0.87 4.21

pi.1<-0.5
lambda.1<-0.09
kappa.1<-1.5
lambda.2<-0.09
kappa.2<-1.5

## True value of the 0.2-quantile of the residual life
## distribution of type 1 event

true.q<-(-(1/lambda.1)*log(1-(1/pi.1)*(pi.1
            xp(-lambda.1*t0^(kappa.1)))
+p*(pi.1*exp(-lambda.1*t0^(kappa.1))+(1-pi.1)*
exp(-lambda.2*t0^(kappa.2))))))))^(1/kappa.1)-t0
```

```
#> true.q
#[1] 2.166371

## Creating Table 4.1

out<-timepoints(xx,unique.1$time)
tbl.1<-round(cbind(unique.1[,c(1,5)],as.
            numeric(out$est[1,]),
as.numeric(out$est[2,]),unique.1[,2]),3)
names(tbl.1)<-c("x","delta","ci.1","ci.2","km")
tbl.1

## Creating Table 4.2

tdiff<-diff(c(0,unique.1$time))
km.new<-c(1,unique.1$km.1.all[1:
            c(length(unique.1$km.1.all)-1)])
tbl.2<-round(cbind(unique.1[,c(1,5,3,6:9)],tdiff,km.new,
                unique.1[,10]),3)
names(tbl.2)<-c("time","event","y","indi.1","indi.2",
                "indi.all","indi.j",
"tdiff","km","incre")
tbl.2[,1:9]

## Creating Figure 4.5

plot(xx,color=c("blue","red"),lty=1:2,xlab="Time",
ylab="Cumulative Incidence Estimates",curvlab=c("Type 1",
                                        "Type 2"))

## Creating Figure 4.6 when sample size=100 (Need to to
## run the above lines after changing the sample size
## to 100

plot(support.points.0,disp.0,type="l",lty=1,
xlab="Support points for 0.2-quantiles",
    ylab="One-sample Statistic")
abline(h=qchisq(0.95,1),lty=2)
```

A.5   Example 4.4 in Sect. 4.4.2

```
## Functions to select a cuminc estimate (Gray) at a fixed
## time x when there are two trt groups and two types
## of events. First subscript is group (0=control;
## 1=active) and second subscript is type of events (1=of
## interest (F1); 2=other (F2))

cuminc.01<-function(x){
max(xx[[1]]$est[xx[[1]]$time <= x])
}
cuminc.11<-function(x){
max(xx[[2]]$est[xx[[2]]$time <= x])
}
cuminc.02<-function(x){
max(xx[[3]]$est[xx[[3]]$time <= x])
}
cuminc.12<-function(x){
max(xx[[4]]$est[xx[[4]]$time <= x])
}


## Functions to select a cuminc estimate (Gray) at a fixed
## time x- when there are two trt groups and two types
## of events. First subscript is group (0=control;
## 1=active) and second subscript is type of events (1=of
## interest (F1); 2=other (F2))

cuminc.01.minus<-function(x){
max(xx[[1]]$est[xx[[1]]$time < x])
}
cuminc.11.minus<-function(x){
max(xx[[2]]$est[xx[[2]]$time < x])
}
cuminc.02.minus<-function(x){
max(xx[[3]]$est[xx[[3]]$time < x])
}
cuminc.12.minus<-function(x){
max(xx[[4]]$est[xx[[4]]$time < x])
}
```

```
## Functions to invert the cuminc estimates (Gray) when
##   there are two groups and two types of events. First
##   subscript is group (0=control;1=active) and second
##   subscript is type of events (1=of interest (F1);
##   2=other (F2))

inv.cuminc.01<-function(x){
min(xx[[1]]$time[xx[[1]]$est >= x])
}
inv.cuminc.11<-function(x){
min(xx[[2]]$time[xx[[2]]$est >= x])
}
inv.cuminc.02<-function(x){
min(xx[[3]]$time[xx[[3]]$est >= x])
}
inv.cuminc.12<-function(x){
min(xx[[4]]$time[xx[[4]]$est >= x])
}


## Data Generation
generate.data<-function(n.obs,pi.1,lambda.1,kappa.1,
                        lambda.2,
kappa.2,cens,group,seed.no)
{
set.seed(seed.no)
binom.number<-rbinom(n.obs,1,pi.1)
u.1<-runif(as.numeric(table(binom.number)[1]),0,1)
u.2<-runif(as.numeric(table(binom.number)[2]),0,1)
time<-rep(NA,n.obs)
time[binom.number==0]<-(-(1/lambda.1)*log(1-u.1))
                       ^(1/kappa.1)
time[binom.number==1]<-(-(1/lambda.2)*log(1-u.2))
                       ^(1/kappa.2)
censored<-runif(n.obs,0,cens)
obs.time<-apply(cbind(time,censored),1,min)
event.i<-rep(NA,n.obs)
event.i[binom.number==0]<-1
event.i[binom.number==1]<-2
event.i[obs.time==censored]<-0
group.i<-rep(group,n.obs) #Defining group
```

```
data.frame(cbind(obs.time,group.i,event.i))
}

temp.0<-generate.data(100,0.5,0.09,1.5,0.09,1.5,45,0,3224)
temp.1<-generate.data(100,0.5,0.09,1.5,0.09,1.5,45,1,7344)

temp<-data.frame(rbind(temp.0,temp.1))
names(temp)<-c("time","group","event")

my.data<-temp[order(temp$time),]

library(cmprsk)
xx <- cuminc(my.data$time,my.data$event,my.data$group)

obs.time<-temp$time
event.i<-temp$event
group.i<-temp$group

## Setting up p-quantile and a fixed time point for
## the residual life distribution

p<-0.2
t0<-2

## How to extract F_1(x), F_1(x-), F_2(x), and F_2(x-) to
## calculate S(x)-S(x-) in control group

time.comb<-sort(obs.time[event.i==1 | event.i==2])
F01.x<-apply(t(time.comb),2,cuminc.01)
F01.x.minus<-apply(t(time.comb),2,cuminc.01.minus)
F02.x<-apply(t(time.comb),2,cuminc.02)
F02.x.minus<-apply(t(time.comb),2,cuminc.02.minus)

F11.x<-apply(t(time.comb),2,cuminc.11)
F11.x.minus<-apply(t(time.comb),2,cuminc.11.minus)
F12.x<-apply(t(time.comb),2,cuminc.12)
F12.x.minus<-apply(t(time.comb),2,cuminc.12.minus)

km1.x<-(1-F01.x-F02.x)
km1.x.minus<-(1-F01.x.minus-F02.x.minus)
```

```
km2.x<-(1-F11.x-F12.x)
km2.x.minus<-(1-F11.x.minus-F12.x.minus)

## Calculating the variance of u.1 in group 1

km.1.t0<-1-cuminc.01(t0)-cuminc.02(t0)
q1.t0<-inv.cuminc.01(cuminc.01(t0)+p*km.1.t0)-t0

temp.surv.1<-survfit(Surv(obs.time[group.i==0],
as.numeric(event.i[group.i==0]>0))~1)
temp.my<-my.data[!is.na(pmatch(round(my.data$time,3),
round(temp.surv.1$time,3))),]

unique.1<-data.frame(cbind(temp.surv.1$time,
                    temp.surv.1$surv,
temp.surv.1$n.risk,temp.surv.1$n.event,temp.my$event))
names(unique.1)<-c("time","km.1.all","y","dN",
                    "event.type")

unique.1$indi.t0.q1.t0<-rep(0,length(unique.1[,1]))
unique.1$indi.t0.q1.t0[unique.1$time >= t0 &
unique.1$time <= t0+q1.t0]<-1

unique.1$indi.0.t0<-rep(0,length(unique.1[,1]))
unique.1$indi.0.t0[unique.1$time > 0 &
unique.1$time <= t0]<-1

unique.1$indi.all.events<-rep(0,length(unique.1[,1]))
unique.1$indi.all.events[unique.1$event.type > 0]<-1

unique.1$indi.event.j<-rep(0,length(unique.1[,1]))
unique.1$indi.event.j[unique.1$event.type == 1]<-1

unique.1$dS.diff<-diff(c(0,unique.1$time))*
c(1,unique.1$km.1.all[1:c(length(unique.1$km.1.all)-1)])

term.1.1<-(unique.1$indi.t0.q1.t0*unique.1$km.1.all*
unique.1$indi.event.j)/unique.1$y
term.1.2<-cumsum((unique.1$indi.t0.q1.t0*
                unique.1$km.1.all*
```

```
unique.1$indi.event.j)/unique.1$y^2)
term.1<-term.1.1-term.1.2

term.2.1<-unique.1$indi.t0.q1.t0*unique.1$dS.diff*
((unique.1$indi.event.j)/unique.1$y)
term.2.2<-unique.1$dS.diff*cumsum(unique.1$indi.t0.q1.t0*
(unique.1$indi.event.j)/unique.1$y^2)
term.2<-term.2.1-term.2.2

term.3.1<-p*km.1.t0*unique.1$indi.0.t0*
(unique.1$indi.all.events/unique.1$y)
term.3.2<-p*km.1.t0*cumsum(unique.1$indi.0.t0*
(unique.1$indi.all.events/unique.1$y^2))
term.3<-term.3.1-term.3.2

var.1<-sum((term.1-term.2-term.3)^2) # variance of u.1
                                     # in group 1


## Calculating the variance of u.2 in group 2

km.2.t0<-1-cuminc.11(t0)-cuminc.12(t0)
q2.t0<-inv.cuminc.11(cuminc.11(t0)+p*km.2.t0)-t0

temp.surv.2<-survfit(Surv(obs.time[group.i==1],
as.numeric(event.i[group.i==1]>0))~1)
temp.my<-my.data[!is.na(pmatch(round(my.data$time,3),
round(temp.surv.2$time,3))),]

unique.2<-data.frame(cbind(temp.surv.2$time,
                    temp.surv.2$surv,
temp.surv.2$n.risk,temp.surv.2$n.event,temp.my$event))
names(unique.2)<-c("time","km.2.all","y","dN",
                "event.type")

unique.2$indi.t0.q2.t0<-rep(0,length(unique.2[,1]))
unique.2$indi.t0.q2.t0[unique.2$time >= t0 &
unique.2$time <= t0+q2.t0]<-1

unique.2$indi.0.t0<-rep(0,length(unique.2[,1]))
unique.2$indi.0.t0[unique.2$time > 0 &
```

```r
unique.2$time <= t0]<-1

unique.2$indi.all.events<-rep(0,length(unique.2[,1]))
unique.2$indi.all.events[unique.2$event.type > 0]<-1

unique.2$indi.event.j<-rep(0,length(unique.2[,1]))
unique.2$indi.event.j[unique.2$event.type == 1]<-1

unique.2$dS.diff<-diff(c(0,unique.2$time))*
c(1,unique.2$km.1.all[1:c(length(unique.2$km.1.all)-1)])

term.1.1<-(unique.2$indi.t0.q2.t0*unique.2$km.2.all*
unique.2$indi.event.j)/unique.2$y
term.1.2<-cumsum((unique.2$indi.t0.q2.t0
                 *unique.2$km.2.all*
unique.2$indi.event.j)/unique.2$y^2)
term.1<-term.1.1-term.1.2

term.2.1<-unique.2$indi.t0.q2.t0*unique.2$dS.diff*
((unique.2$indi.event.j)/unique.2$y)
term.2.2<-unique.2$dS.diff*cumsum(unique.2$indi.t0.q2.t0*
(unique.2$indi.event.j)/unique.2$y^2)
term.2<-term.2.1-term.2.2

term.3.1<-p*km.1.t0*unique.2$indi.0.t0*
(unique.2$indi.all.events/unique.2$y)
term.3.2<-p*km.1.t0*cumsum(unique.2$indi.0.t0*
(unique.2$indi.all.events/unique.2$y^2))
term.3<-term.3.1-term.3.2

var.2<-sum((term.1-term.2-term.3)^2) # variance of u.2
                                     # in group 2
eta<-seq(0.0,4.0,0.01)
time.minimax<-min(max(obs.time[group.i==0]),
max(obs.time[group.i==1]))
support.points<-seq(0,time.minimax,0.01)
term.1<-apply(as.matrix(support.points),1,
function(x){(cuminc.01(t0+x)-cuminc.01(t0)-p*km.1.t0)^2
             /var.1})
```

```
support.matrix.group2<-apply(as.matrix(eta),1,
function(x){x*support.points})
min.dispersion.eta<-apply(support.matrix.group2,2,
function(x){
term.2<-apply(as.matrix(x),1,function(x){
(cuminc.11(t0+x)-cuminc.11(t0)-p*km.2.t0)^2/var.2})
support.limit<-min(length(term.1),length(term.2))
test.stat<-cbind(support.points[1:support.limit],
term.1[1:support.limit]+term.2[1:support.limit])
min.rows<-as.numeric(test.stat[test.stat[,2]==
min(test.stat[,2]),])
min.rows[length(min.rows)]
})


covered.eta<-eta[min.dispersion.eta < qchisq(0.95,1)]

## 95% confidence interval for the ratio of two
## 0.2-quantile residual lifetimes of type 1 events

c(min(covered.eta),max(covered.eta))
# [1] 0.44 2.93

## Value of the two-sample statistic under the null
## hypothesis
min.dispersion.eta[eta==1]
#[1] 0.02063819

## Creating Figure 4.7

plot(eta,min.dispersion.eta,type="l",lty=1,
xlab="Ratio of two 0.2-quantiles",
ylab="Two-sample Statistic")
abline(h=qchisq(0.95,1),lty=2)

## 0.2-quantile residual lifetime for group 0
q1.t0
#[1] 2.361196
```

```
## 0.2-quantile residual lifetime for group 1
q2.t0
#[1] 2.341192
```

A.6   Example 5.2 in Sect. 5.2.3

```
library(emplik)

fun<-function(t){t}
maxit<-25
mu<-3.5

## Mock dataset
x <- c(1, 1.5, 2, 3, 4, 5, 6, 5, 4, 1, 2, 4.5)
d <- c(1,   1, 0, 1, 0, 1, 1, 1, 1, 0, 0,   1)

xvec <- as.vector(x)
nn <- length(xvec)
temp <- Wdataclean2(xvec, d)
x <- temp$value
d <- temp$dd
w <- temp$weight
xd1 <- x[d == 1]
funxd1 <- fun(xd1)
xd0 <- x[d == 0]
wd1 <- w[d == 1]
wd0 <- w[d == 0]
m <- length(xd0)

## Empirical likelihood under the general constraint
## (under H_1)
temp3 <- WKM(x = x, d = d, w = w) # Yields the same
                                  # results from survfit
logel00 <- temp3$logel
logel00
#[1] -16.42593

## One step estimates of p_j
```

```
pnew <- el.test.wt(x = funxd1, wt = wd1, mu = mu)$prob
n <- length(pnew)
k <- rep(NA, m)
for (i in 1:m) { # Generate positions censored
                  observations+1
     k[i] <- 1 + n - sum(xd1 > xd0[i])
}


## Constrained EM algorithm
num <- 1
while (num < maxit) {
    wd1new <- wd1
    sur <- rev(cumsum(rev(pnew)))
        for (i in 1:m) {
            wd1new[k[i]:n] <- wd1new[k[i]:n] + wd0[i] *
                              pnew[k[i]:n]/sur[k[i]]
        }
    temp9 <- el.test.wt(funxd1, wt = wd1new, mu)
    pnew <- temp9$prob
    lam <- temp9$lam
    num <- num + 1
    }
sur <- rev(cumsum(rev(pnew)))


## Final estimates of p_j
pnew
#[1] 0.1489836 0.1516380 0.1447664 0.1108301 0.1277623
     0.2251085 0.0909112


## Survival probability estimates based on final estimates
    of p_j
sur[k]
#[1] 0.8510164 0.6993784 0.4437820


## Empirical likelihood under H_0
logel <- sum(wd1 * log(pnew)) + sum(wd0 * log(sur[k]))
logel
#[1] -17.04924
```

```
## Empirical log-likelihood ratio
2 * (logel00 - logel)
#[1] 1.246634
```

References

[1] Aalen, O. O. (1975). Statistical inference for a family of counting processes. Ph.D. Dissertation, University of California, Berkeley.

[2] Aalen, O. O. (1978). Nonparametric inference for a family of counting processes. *Annals of Statistics* **6**, 701–726.

[3] Alam, K. and Kulasekera, K. B. (1993). Estimation of the quantile function of residual life time distribution. *Journal of Statistical Planning and Inference* **37**, 327–337.

[4] Aly, E. A. A. (1992). On some confidence bands for percentile residual life functions. *Nonparametric statistics* **2**, 59–70.

[5] Andersen, P. K., Borgan, Ø., Gill, R. D. and Keiding, N. (1993). *Statistical Models Based on Counting Processes.* New York: Springer-Verlag.

[6] Arnold, B. C. and Brockett, P. L. (1983). When does the βth percentile residual life function determine the distribution. *Operations Research* **31**, 391–396.

[7] Bandos, H. (2007). Regression on median residual life function for censored survival data. Ph.D. Dissertation, University of Pittsburgh.

J.-H. Jeong, *Statistical Inference on Residual Life*,
Statistics for Biology and Health, DOI 10.1007/978-1-4939-0005-3,
© Springer Science+Business Media New York 2014

182   *REFERENCES*

[8] Barabas, B., Csörgö, M., Horvath, L. and Yandell, B. S. (1986). Bootstrapped confidence bands for percentile lifetime. *Annals of the Institute of Statistical Mathematics* **38**, 429–438.

[9] Bahadur, R. R. (1966). A note on quantiles in large samples. *Annals of Mathematical Statistics* **37**, 577–580.

[10] Bartholomew, D. J. (1973). *Stochastic Models for Social Processes.* Second Edition. New York: Wiley & Sons.

[11] Basawa, I. V. and Koul, H. L. (1988). Large-sample statistics based on quadratic dispersion. *International Statistical Review* **56**, 199–219.

[12] Bauer, H. (1995). *Probability Theory.* Berlin: Walter de Gruyter & Co.

[13] Berger, R. L., Boos, D. D. and Guess, F. M. (1988). Tests and confidence sets for comparing two mean residual life functions. *Biometrics* **44**, 103–115.

[14] Beyersmann, J., Dettenkofer, M., Bertz, H. and Schumacher, M. (2007). A competing risks analysis of blood stream infection after stem-cell transplantation using subdistribution hazards and cause-specific hazards. *Statistics in Medicine* **26**, 5360–5369.

[15] Beyersmann, J., Latouche, A., Buchholz, A. and Schumacher, M. (2009). Simulating competing risks data in survival analysis. *Statistics in Medicine* **28**, 956–971.

[16] Berger, R. L., Boos, D. D. and Guess, F. M.(1988). Tests and confidence sets for comparing two mean residual life functions. *Biometrics* **44**, 103–115.

[17] Bhattacharjee, M. C. (1982). The class of mean residual lives and some consequences. *SIAM J. Algebraic Discrete Methods* **3**, 56–65.

[18] Borel, E. (1909). Les probabilités dénombrables et leurs applications arithmetiques. *Rend. Circ. Mat. Palermo* **27**, 247–271.

[19] Bryson, M. C. and Siddiqui, M. M. (1969). Soma criteria for aging. *Journal of American Statistical Association* **64**, 1472–1483.

[20] Buckley, J. J. and James, I. R. (1979). Linear regression with censored data. *Biometrika* **66**, 429–436.

[21] Cajori, F. (1911). Historical Note on the Newton-Raphson Method of Approximation. *The American Mathematical Monthly* **18**, 29–32.

[22] Cantelli, F. P. (1917). Sulla probabilità come limite della frequenza. *Atti Accad. Naz. Lincei* **26**, 39–45.

[23] Cantelli, F. P. (1933). Sulla determinazione empirica delle leggi di probabilita. *Giorn. Ist. Ital. Attuari* **4**, 221–424.

[24] Chan, K. C. G., Chen, Y. Q. and Di, C.-Z. (2012). Proportional mean residual life model for right-censored length-biased data. *Biometrika*, doi:10.1093/biomet/ass049.

[25] Chen, X. and Wang, Q. (2013). Semiparametric mean residual life model with covariates missing at random. *Journal of Nonparametric Statistics*, **25**, 647–663.

[26] Chen, Y. Q. (2007). Additive expectancy regression. *Journal of the American Statistical Association* **102**, 153–166.

[27] Chen, Y. Q. and Cheng, S. (2005). Semiparametric regression analysis of mean residual life with censored survival data. *Biometrika* **92**, 19–29.

[28] Chen, Y. Q. and Cheng, S. (2006). Linear life expectancy regression with censored data. *Biometrika* **93**, 303–313.

[29] Chen, Y. Q., Jewell, N. P., Lei, X. and Cheng, S. C. (2005). Semiparametric estimation of proportional mean residual life model in presence of censoring. *Biometrics* **61**, 170–178.

[30] Chen, Y.-Y., Hollander, M. and Langberg, N. A. (1983). Tests for monotone mean residual life, using randomly censored data. *Biometrics* **39**, 119–127.

[31] Chiang, C. L. (1968). *Introduction to Stochastic Processes in Biostatistics.* New York: Wiley.

[32] Chung, C. F. (1989). Confidence bands for percentile residual lifetime under random censorship model. *Journal of Multivariate Analysis* **29**, 94–126.

[33] Cox, D. R. (1962). *Renewal Theory.* London: Methuen.

[34] Cox, D. R. (1972). Regression models and life-tables. *Journal of the Royal Statistical Society-Series B* **34**, 187–220.

[35] Cox, D. R. (1975). Partial likelihood. *Biometrika* **62**, 269–276.

[36] Cox, D. R. and Oakes, D. (1984). *Analysis of Survival Data.* London: Chapman & Hall.

[37] Csörgö, M. (1983). Quantile processes with statistical applications. Regional Conference Series in Applied Mathematics, SIAM, Philadelphia.

[38] Csörgö, M., and Csörgö, S. (1987). Estimation of percentile residual life. *Operations Research* **35**, 598–606.

[39] Csörgö, M., Csörgö, S. and Horváth, L. (1986). *An Asymptotic Theory for Empirical Reliability and Concentration Processes. Lecture Notes in Statistics* **33**. Berlin: Springer.

[40] Csörgö, S. and Viharos, L. (1992). Confidence bands for percentile residual lifetimes *Journal of Statistical Planning and Inference* **30**, 327–337.

[41] Dabrowska, D. M. and Doksum, K. A. (1998). Estimation and testing in a two-sample generalized odds-rate model. *Journal of the American Statistical Association* **83**, 744–749.

[42] Dasu, T. (1991). The proportional mean residual life model. Ph.D. thesis, University of Rochester.

[43] David, H. and Moeschberger, M. L. (1978). *The Theory of Competing Risks*. London: Griffin.

[44] Deevey, E. S. (1947). Life tables for natura populations of animals. *Quarterly Review of Biology* **22**, 283–314.

[45] Doob, J. L. (1949). Heuristic approach to the Kolmogorov-Smirnov theorems. *Annals of Mahematical Statistics* **20**, 393–403.

[46] Donsker, M. D. (1951). An invariance principle for certain probability limit theorems. *Mem. Am. Math. Soc.* **6**, 1–12.

[47] Durrett, R. (1991). *Probability: Theory and Examples*. Belmont: Wadsworth, Inc.

[48] Escobar, M. D. (1994). Estimating normal means with a Dirichlet process prior. *Journal of the American Statistical Association* **89**, 268–277.

[49] Escobar, M. D. and West, M. (1995). Bayesian density estimation and inference using mixtures. *Journal of the American Statistical Association* **90**, 577–588.

[50] Ferguson, T. S. (1973). A Bayesian analysis of some non-parametric problems. *Annals of Statistics* **1**, 209–230.

[51] Ferguson, T. S. (1974). Prior distributions on spaces of probability measures. *Annals of Statistics* **2**, 615–629.

[52] Fine, J. P. and Gray, R. J. (1999). A proportional hazards model for the subdistribution of a competing risk. *Journal of the American Statistical Association* **94**, 496–509.

[53] Fine, J. P., Jiang, H. and Chappell, R. (2001). On semi-competing risks data. *Biometrika* **88**, 907–919.

[54] Fisher, B., Jeong, J.-H., Anderson, S. *et al.* (2002). Twenty-five year findings from a randomized clinical trial comparing radical mastectomy with total mastectomy and with total mastectomy followed by radiation therapy. *The New England Journal Of Medicine* **347**, 567–575.

[55] Fleming, T. R. and Harrington, D. (1991). *Counting Processes and Survival Analysis*. New York: John Wiley and Sons.

[56] Fligner, M. A. and Rust, S. W. (1982). A modification of Mood's median test for the generalized Behrens-Fisher problem. *Biometrika* **69**, 221–226.

[57] Franco-Pereira, A. M., Lillo, R. E. and Romo, J. (2012). Comparing quantile residual life functions by confidence bands. *Lifetime Data Analysis* **18**, 195–214.

[58] Gâteaux, R. (1913). Sur les fonctionnelles continues et les fonctionnelles analytiques. *Comptes rendus hebdomadaires des séances de l'Académie des sciences (Paris)* **157**, 325–327.

[59] Gâteaux, R. (1919). Fonctions d'une infinité de variables indépendantes. *Bulletin de la Société Mathématique de France* **47**, 70–96.

[60] Gaynor, J. J, Feuer, E. J., Tan, C. C., *et al.* (1993). On the use of cause-specific failure and conditional failure probabilities: Examples from clinical oncology data. *Journal of American Statistical Association* **88**, 400–409.

[61] Gelfand, A. E. and Kottas, A. (2002). A computational approach for full nonparametric Bayesian inference under Dirichlet process mixture models. *The Journal of Computational and Graphical Statistics* **11**, 289–305.

[62] Gelfand, A. E. and Kottas, A. (2003). Bayesian semiparametric regression for median residual life. *Scandinavian Journal of Statistics* **30**, 651–665.

[63] Gertsbakh, I. P. and Kordonskiy, K. B. (1969). *Models of Failure*. New York: Springer-Verlag.

[64] Ghosh, J. K. and Mustafi C. K. (1986). A note on the residual median process. *The Canadian Journal of Statistics* **14**, 251–255.

[65] Glivenko, V. (1933). Sulla determinazione empirica della legge di probabilita. *Giorn. Ist. Ital. Attuari* **4**, 92–99.

[66] Gompertz, B. (1825). On the nature of the function expressive of the law of human mortality, and on the new mode of determining the value of life contingencies. *Phil. Trans. R. Soc. A* **115**, 513–580.

[67] Gray, R. J. (1988). A class of K-sample tests for comparing the cumulative incidence of a competing risk. *Annals of Statistics* **16**, 1141–1154.

[68] Greenwood, M. (1926). The natural duration of cancer. In *Florida State University Statistics Report M4702*, 1–17.

[69] Guess, F. and Proschan, F. (1985). Mean Residual Life: Theory and Application. In *Reports on Public Health and Medical Subjects 33*. London: His Majesty's Stationary Office, 1–26.

[70] Gumbel, E. I. (1924). Eine Darstellung der Sterbetafel. *Biometrika* **16**, 283–96.

[71] Gupta, R. C. and Langford, E. S. (1984). On the determination of a distribution by its median residual life function: a functional equation. *Journal of Applied Probability* **21**, 120–128.

[72] Haile, S. R. (2008). Inference on competing risks in breast cancer data. Ph.D. Dissertation, University of Pittsburgh.

[73] Haines, A. L. and Singpurwalla, N. D. (1974). Some contributions to the stochastic characterization of wear. In *Reliability and Biometry*, 47–80, F. Proschan and R. J. Serfling (eds.) Philadelphia: SIAM.

[74] Hall, P. and La Scala, B. (1990). Methodology and algorithms of empirical likelihood. *International Statistical Review* **58**, 109–127.

[75] Hall, W. J. and Wellner, J. A. (1981). Mean residual life. In *Statistics and Related Topics*, 169–184, M. Csörgö, D.A. Dawson, J. N. K. Rao,and A. K. Md. E. Saleh (eds.) New York: North Holland.

[76] Hollander, M. and Proschan, F. (1975). Tests for the mean residual life. In *Florida State University Statistics Report M326*, 1–19.

[77] Ishwaran, H. and James, L. F. (2001). Gibbs sampling methods for stick-breaking priors. *Journal of the American Statistical Association* **96**, 161–173.

[78] Jeong, J. and Fine, J. P. (2006). Direct parametric inference for cumulative incidence function. *Journal of the Royal Statistical Society-Series C* **55**, 187–200.

[79] Jeong, J. and Fine, J. P. (2007). Parametric regression on cumulative incidence function. *Biostatistics* **8**, 184–196.

[80] Jeong, J. and Fine, J. P. (2009). A note on cause-specific residual life. *Biometrika* **96**, 237–242.

[81] Jeong, J. and Fine, J. P. (2013). Nonparametric inference on cause-specific quantile residual life. *Biometrical Journal* **55**, 68–81.

[82] Jeong, J., Jung, S. and Costantino, J. P. (2007). Nonparametric inference on median residual life function. *Biometrics* **64**, 157–163.

[83] Joe, H. (1985). Characterizations of life distributions from percentile residual lifetimes. *Annals of the Institute of Statistical Mathematics* **37**, 165–172.

[84] Joe, H. and Proschan, F. (1984). Percentile residual life functions. *Operations Research* **32**, 668–678.

[85] Jung, S., Jeong, J. and Bandos, H. (2009). Regression on quantile residual life *Biometrics* **65**, 1203–1212.

[86] Kalbfleisch, J. D. and Prentice, R. L. (1980). *The Statistical Analysis of Failure Time Data.* New York: John Wiley & Sons.

[87] Kalbfleisch, J. D. and Prentice, R. L. (2002). *The Statistical Analysis of Failure Time Data.* Second Edition. New Jersey: John Wiley and Sons, Inc.

[88] Kaplan, E. P. and Meier, P. (1958). Nonparametric estimation from incomplete observations. *Journal of the American Statistical Association* **53**, 457–481.

[89] Karlin, S. and Taylor, H. M. (1975). *A First Course in Stochastic Processes.* Second Edition. San Diego: Academic Press, Inc.

[90] Katsahian, S., Resche-Rigon, M., Chevret, S. and Porcher, R. (2006). Analysing multicentre competing risks data with a mixed proportional hazards model for the subdistribution. *Statistics in Medicine* **25**, 4267–4278.

[91] Kim, M. and Yang, Y. (2011). Semiparametric approach to a random effects quantile regression model. *Journal of the American Statistical Association* **106**, 1405–1417.

[92] Kim, M., Zhou, M. and Jeong, J. (2012). Censored quantile regression for residual lifetimes. *Lifetime Data Analysis* **18**, 177–194.

[93] Koenker, R. and Bassett, G. (1978). Regression quantiles. *Econometrica* **46**, 33–50.

[94] Korn, E. L. and Dorey, F. J. (1992). Applications of crude incidence curves. *Statististics in Medicine* **11**, 813–829.

[95] Kottas, A. (2006). Nonparametric Bayesian survival analysis using mixtures of Weibull distributions. *Journal of Statistical Planning and Inference* **136**, 578–596.

[96] Kottas, A. and Gelfand, A. E. (2001). Bayesian semiparametric median regression modeling. *Journal of the American Statistical Association* **96**, 1458–1468.

[97] Koul, H., Susarla, V. and Van Ryzin, J. (1981). Least squares regression analysis with censored survival data. In *Topics in Applied Statistics*, 151–165, Y. P. Chaubey and T. D. Dwivedi (eds.) New York: Marcel Dekker.

[98] Lagrange, J.-L. (1806). *Leons sur le calcul des fonctions.* (in French). Courcier.

[99] Lillo, R. E. (2005). On the median residual lifetime and its aging properties: a characterization theorem and its applications. *Naval Research Logistics* **52**, 370–380.

[100] Lim, J. (2011). Inference on censored survival data under competing risks. Ph.D. Dissertation, University of Pittsburgh.

[101] Lin, D. Y. (1997). Non-parametric inference for cumulative incidence functions in competing risks studies. *Statististics in Medicine* **16**, 901–910.

[102] Liu, S. and Ghosh, S. (2008). Regression analysis of mean residual life function. *Institute of Statistical Mimeo Series #2613*, North Carolina State University, Raleigh.

[103] López-Pintado, S. and Romo, J. (2009). On the concept of depth for functional data. *Journal of the American Statistical Association* **104**, 718–734.

[104] Ma, Y. and Yin, G. (2009). Semiparametric median residual life model and inference. *The Canadian Journal of Statistics* **34**, 665–679.

[105] Ma, Y. and Wei, Y. (2012). Analysis on censored quantile residual life model via spline smoothing. *Statistica Sinica* **22**, 47–68.

[106] Maguluri, G. and Zhang, C. H. (1994). Estimation in the mean residual life regression-model. *Journal of the Royal Statistical Society Series-B* **56**, 477–489.

[107] McLain, A. C. Ghosh, S. K. (2011). Nonparametric estimation of the conditional mean residual life function with censored data. *Lifetime Data Analysis* **17**, 514–532.

[108] Morrison, D. G. and Schmittlein, D. C. (1980). Strikes and wars: probability models for duration. *Organizational Behavior and Human Performance* **25**, 224–251.

[109] Mute, E. J. (1977). Reliability models with positive memory derived from the mean residual life function. In *Theory and Applications of Reliability*, Tsokos, C. P. and Shimi, I. N. (eds.) New York: Academic Press.

[110] Nair, K. R. M and·Nair, N. U. (1989). Bivariate mean residual life. *IEEE Transactions on Reliability* **38**, 362–364.

[111] Nelson, W. (1972). Theory and applications of hazard plotting for censored failure data. *Technometrics* **14**, 945–965.

[112] Oakes, D. and Dasu, T. (1990). A note on residual life (with discussion). *Biometrika* **77**, 409–410.

[113] Oakes, D. and Dasu, T. (2003). Inference for the proportional mean residual life model. *The Institute of Mathematical Statistics Lecture Notes-Monograph Series* **43**, 105–116.

[114] Owen, A. B. (1988). Empirical likelihood ratio confidence intervals for a single functional. *Biometrika* **75**, 237–249.

[115] Owen, A. B. (1990). Empirical likelihood ratio confidence regions. *The Annals of Statistics* **18**, 90–120.

[116] Owen, A. B. (2001). *Empirical Likelihood*. Boca Raton: Chapman & Hall/CRC.

[117] Park, T., Jeong, J. and Lee, J. (2012). Nonparametric Bayesian inference on quantile residual life function. *Statistics in Medicine* **31**, 1972–1985.

[118] Peng, L. and Fine, J. P. (2007). Nonparametric quantile inference with competing risks data. *Biometrika* **94**, 735–744.

[119] Pepe, M. S. (1991). Inference for events with dependent risks in multiple endpoint studies. *Journal of the American Statistical Association* **86**, 770–778.

[120] Pepe, M. S. and Mori, M. (1993). Kaplan-Meier, marginal or conditional probability curves in summarizing competing risks failure time data? *Statistics in Medicine* **12**, 737–751.

[121] Peto, R. and Peto, J. (1972). Asymptotically efficient rank invariant test procedures (with discussion). *Journal of the Royal Statistical Society-Series A* **135**, 185–206.

[122] Pintilie, M. (2006). *Competing Risks: A Practical Perspective*. Chichester: John Wiley & Sons, Ltd.

[123] Prentice, R. L., Kalbeisch, J. D., Peterson, Jr., A. V., Flournoy, N., Farewell, V. T. and Breslow, N. E. (1978). The analysis of failure times in the presence of competing risks. *Biometrics* **34**, 541–554.

[124] Pyke, R. (1965). Spacings (with discussion). *Journal of the Royal Statistical Society Series B* **27**, 395–449.

[125] R Development Core Team (2008). R: A language and environment for statistical computing. R Foundation for Statistical Computing, Vienna, Austria. ISBN 3-900051-07-0, URL http://www.R-project.org.

[126] Rao, B. R., Damaraju, C. V. and Alhumoud, J. M. (1993). Covariate effect on the life expectancy and percentile residual life functions under the proportional hazards and the accelerated life models. *Communication in Statistics: Theory and Methods* **22**, 257–281.

[127] Ross, S. M. (1985). *Introduction to Probability Models*. Third Edition. Orlando: Academic Press, Inc.

[128] Rotnitzky, A. and Robins, J. M. (2005). Inverse Probability Weighted Estimation in Survival Analysis. *Encyclopedia of Biostatistics*.

[129] Schmittlein, D. C. and Morrison, D. G. (1981). The median residual lifetime: a characterization theorem and application. *Operations Research* **29**, 392–399.

[130] Shorack, G. R. and Wellner, J. A. (2009). *Empirical Processes with Applications to Statistics*. The SIAM edition. Philadelphia: John Wiley & Sons, Inc.

[131] Shi, H., Cheng, Y. and Jeong, J. (2013). Constrained parametric regression on cumulative incidence functions. *Biometrical Journal* **55**, 82–96.

[132] Slutsky, E. (1925). Über stochastische Asymptoten und Grenzwerte. *Metron* (in German) **5**, 3–89.

[133] Song, J. and Cho, G. (1995). A note on percentile residual life. *Sankhya* **57**, 333–335.

[134] Stute, W. (1996). Distributional convergence under random censorship when covariates are present. *Scandinavian Journal of Statistics* **23**, 461–471.

[135] Su, J. Q. and Wei, L. J. (1993). Nonparametric estimation for the difference or ratio of median failure times. *Biometrics* **49**, 603–607.

[136] Sun, L., Song, X. and Zhang, Z. (2011). Mean residual life models with time-dependent coefficients under right censoring. *Biometrika* **99**, 185–197.

[137] Sun, L. and Zhang, Z. (2009). A class of transformed mean residual life models with censored survival data. *Journal of the American Statistical Association* **104**, 803–815.

[138] Thomas, D. R. and Grunkemeier, G. L. (1975). Confidence interval estimation of survival probabilities for censored data. *Journal of the American Statistical Association* **70**, 865–871.

[139] Tukey, J. W. (1977). *Exploratory Data Analysis* (1970–71: preliminary edition). Reading: Addison-Wesley.

[140] Turnbull, B. (1976). The empirical distribution function with arbitrarily grouped, censored and truncated data. *Journal of the Royal Statistical Society-Series B* **38**, 290–295.

[141] van der Laan, M. and Robins, J. M. (2003). *Unified Methods for Censored Longitudinal Data and Causality*. New York: Springer.

[142] van Dyk, D. and Park, T. (2008). Partially collapsed Gibbs samplers: theory and methods. *Journal of the American Statistical Association* **103**, 790–796.

[143] Wang, J. L. and Hettmansperger, T. P. (1990). Two-sample inference for median survival times based on one sample procedures for censored survival data. *Journal of the American Statistical Association* **85**, 529–536.

[144] Watson, G. S. and Wells, W. T. (1961). On the possibility of improving the meanuseful life of items by eliminating those with short lives. *Technometrics* **3**, 281–298.

[145] Wei, L. J., Ying, Z. and Lin, D. Y. (1990). Linear regression analysis of censored survival data based on rank tests. *Biometrika* **19**, 845–851.

[146] Williams, D. (1991). *Probability with Martingales*. Cambridge University Press.

[147] Xie J. and Liu C. (2005). Adjusted Kaplan-Meier estimator and log-rank test with inverse probability of treatment weighting for survival data. *Statistics in Medicine* **24**, 3089–3110.

[148] Yang, G. (1978). Estimation of a biometric function. *Annals of Statistics* **6**, 112–16.

[149] Ying, Z., Jung, S. and Wei, L. J. (1995). Survival analysis with median regression models. *Journal of the American Statistical Association* **90**,178–184.

[150] Zhao, Y. and Qin, G. (2006). Inference for the mean residual life function via empirical likelihood. *Communications in Statistics - Theory and Methods* **35**, 1025–1036.

[151] Zhang, Z., Zhao, X. and Sun, L. (2010). Goodness-of-fit tests for additive mean residual life model under right censoring. *Lifetime Data Analysis* **16**, 385–408.

[152] Zhou, M. (2005). Empirical likelihood ratio with arbitrarily censored/truncated data by EM algorithm. *Journal of Computational and Graphical Statistics* **14**, 643–656.

[153] Zhou, M., and Jeong, J. (2011). Empirical likelihood ratio test for median and mean residual lifetime. *Statistics in Medicine* **30**, 152–159.

[154] Zhou, M., Kim, M. and Bathke, C. (2012). Empirical likelihood analysis for the heteroscedastic accelerated failure time model. *Statistica Sinica* **22**, 295–316.

About the Author

Dr. Jong-Hyeon Jeong is a full professor of Biostatistics at the University of Pittsburgh. Dr. Jeong's main research area has been survival analysis and clinical trials. In survival analysis, he has worked on frailty modeling, efficiency of survival probability estimates from the proportional hazards model, weighted log-rank test, competing risks, quantile residual life, and likelihood theory such as empirical likelihood and hierarchical likelihood. In clinical trials, he has been involved in several phase III clinical trials on breast cancer treatment as the primary statistician. He has been teaching statistical theory courses and survival analysis in the Department of Biostatistics at the University of Pittsburgh. Dr. Jeong holds his Ph.D. degree in statistics from the University of Rochester and has been an elected member of the International Statistical Institute (ISI) since 2007.

J.-H. Jeong, *Statistical Inference on Residual Life*,
Statistics for Biology and Health, DOI 10.1007/978-1-4939-0005-3,
© Springer Science+Business Media New York 2014

Index

J.-H. Jeong, *Statistical Inference on Residual Life*,
Statistics for Biology and Health, DOI 10.1007/978-1-4939-0005-3,
© Springer Science+Business Media New York 2014

Printed by Publishers' Graphics LLC
JCIMO140131.17.00.10